From The Eating Disorders Program at
THE HOSPITAL FOR SICK CHILDREN

Help for
Eating
Disorders

A Parent's Guide to Symptoms, Causes & Treatments

Dr. Debra K. Katzman, MD, FRCP(C)
& Dr. Leora Pinhas, MD, FRCP(C)

Robert
ROSE

DEDICATION

To my family, my husband, Bob, and my children, Jonathan and Amy,
thank you for your love, support, and encouragement.
— *Debra K. Katzman*

To my father, Albert Pinhas, who inspired me, and to my partner, Steven Lewis,
who has always supported me unconditionally.
— *Leora Pinhas*

The editors would to thank The Hospital for Sick Children and Robert Rose Inc. for giving us the opportunity to create a practical book for parents incorporating the best up-to-date information on treatment with our model of interdisciplinary collaborative care.

This book is a general guide only and should never be a substitute for the skill, knowledge, and experience of a qualified medical professional dealing with the facts, circumstances, and symptoms of a particular case.

The nutritional, medical, and health information presented in this book is based on the research, training, and professional experience of the authors, and is true and complete to the best of their knowledge. However, this book is intended only as an informative guide for those wishing to know more about health, nutrition, and medicine; it is not intended to replace or countermand the advice given by the reader's personal physician. Because each person and situation is unique, the authors and the publisher urge the reader to check with a qualified health-care professional before using any procedure where there is a question as to its appropriateness. A physician should be consulted before beginning any exercise program. The author and the publisher are not responsible for any adverse effects or consequences resulting from the use of the information in this book. It is the responsibility of the reader to consult a physician or other qualified health-care professional regarding personal care.

**Library and Archives Canada
Cataloguing in Publication**

Katzman, Debra
   Help for eating disorders : a parents' guide to symptoms, causes & treatments / Debra Katzman and Leora Pinhas.

Includes index.
ISBN 0-7788-0115-2

1. Eating disorders in children. 2. Eating disorders in adolescence. I. Pinhas, Leora II. Title.

RJ506.E18K38 2005   618.92'8526   C2004-906542-4

Printed and bound in Canada.

1 2 3 4 5 6 7 8 9 CPL 13 12 11 10 09 08 07 06 05

Edited by Bob Hilderley, Senior Editor, Health.

Copyedited by Fina Scroppo.

Design and page composition
   by PageWave Graphics Inc.

Illustrations on pages 48 and 52
   by Crowle Art Group.

The publisher acknowledges the financial support of the Government of Canada through the Book Publishing Industry Development Program.

Published by Robert Rose Inc.,
120 Eglinton Ave. E., Suite 800,
Toronto, Ontario, Canada M4P 1E2
Tel: (416) 322-6552 Fax: (416) 322-6936

Contents

Contributors

PART 1 Diagnosing Eating Disorders

What Is an Eating Disorder?
Debra K. Katzman, MD, FRCP(C),
and Leora Pinhas, MD, FRCP(C)

What Are the Myths and Misconceptions about Eating Disorders?
Ahmed Boachie, MB, ChB, MRCPsych, DCH,
FRCP(C), and Karin Jasper, PhD, MEd

Who Is at Risk for Developing an Eating Disorder?
Debra K. Katzman, MD, FRCP(C),
and Lily Cugliari-Kobayashi, RN, PCN/NP,
HTCP (Level III)

What Factors Cause the Increasing Prevalence of Eating Disorders?
Karin Jasper, PhD, Med, and Ahmed Boachie,
MB, ChB, MRCPsych, DCH, FRCP(C)

What Is Normal Adolescent Development?
Eudice Goldberg, MD, FRCP(C), Gad Reisler,
MD, and Nogah Kerem, MD

How Do You Identify a Child or Adolescent with an Eating Disorder?
Karen Leslie, MD, FRCP(C),
and Anganette Hall, MBChB, DCH

What Are the Possible Medical Complications of Eating Disorders?
Natasha Johnson-Ramgeet, MD, FRCP(C)

What Is My Child Thinking?
Clare Roscoe, MD, FRCP(C)

How Could This Have Happened to Our Family? • *A Mother's Story*
Susan Bauman-Fenicky

PART 2 Treating Eating Disorders

Charting the Road to Recovery
Margus Heinmaa, MPsy, PhD Candidate

Exploring Treatment Resources in Your Community
Donna Samuels, RN, and Heather Graham,
BSc (Psych)

Getting an Assessment
Patti Schabas, MD, FRCP(C)

Choosing a Treatment Strategy
Pier Bryden, M.Phil, MD, FRCP(C)

Learning to Eat Again
Kelly Sherwood, RD, Tania Turrini, RD,
and Kellie Welch, RD

Coping with Lapses and Relapses
Caitlin Shipley, MSW, RSW

Making the Transition from the Adolescent to the Adult Treatment System
Blake Woodside, MD, and Gina Dimitropoulos,
MSW, RSW, PhD Candidate

The Struggle of My Life • *A Patient's Story*
Tammy Balaban

PART 3 Family and Community Roles in Recovery and Prevention

Everyone Needs Help
Geordie Colvin, MSW, RSW

Helping Yourself to Help Your Child
Sheila Bjarnason, MSW, RSW

Looking for Help from Friends
Elise Byer, MSW, RSW

Preventing Eating Disorders by Educating Teachers, Coaches, and Counselors
Gail McVey, PhD, C Psych

Understanding the Long and Hard Journey to Recovery
Max Figueroa, MD and Debra K. Katzman, MD,
FRCP(C)

Eating Disorder Information Resources
Debra K. Katzman, MD, FRCP(C),
and Leora Pinhas, MD, FRCP(C)

Credentials & Affiliations

Ahmed Boachie, MB, ChB, MRCPsych, DCH, FRCP(C)
Child and Adolescent Psychiatrist, The Eating Disorders Program

Lecturer, Department of Psychiatry, Child and Adolescent Psychiatry and Women's Mental Health, The Hospital for Sick Children and University of Toronto

Sheila Bjarnason, MSW, RSW
The Eating Disorders Program, The Hospital for Sick Children

Pier Bryden, M.Phil, MD, FRCP(C)
Lecturer, Department of Psychiatry, Director of Postgraduate Education, Department of Psychiatry, The Hospital for Sick Children and University of Toronto

Elise Byer, MSW, RSW
The Eating Disorders Program, The Hospital for Sick Children

Geordie Colvin, MSW, RSW
The Eating Disorders Day Hospital, The Hospital for Sick Children

Lily Cugliari-Kobayashi, RN, PCN/NP, HTCP (Level III)
The Eating Disorders Day Hospital, The Hospital for Sick Children

Gina Dimitropoulos, MSW, RSW, PhD Candidate
Clinical Social Worker, Inpatient Eating Disorder Program, University Health Network, Toronto General Hospital

Max Figueroa, MD
Clinical Fellow, Division of Adolescent Medicine, Department of Paediatrics, The Hospital for Sick Children and University of Toronto

Eudice Goldberg, MD, FRCP(C)
Associate Professor of Paediatrics, Division of Adolescent Medicine, Department of Paediatrics, The Hospital for Sick Children and University of Toronto

Heather Graham, BSc (Psych)
Intake Coordinator, The Eating Disorders Program, The Hospital for Sick Children

Anganette Hall, MBChB, DCH
Clinical Fellow, Division of Adolescent Medicine, Department of Paediatrics, The Hospital for Sick Children and University of Toronto

Margus Heinmaa, MPsy, PhD Candidate
Pre-Doctoral Fellow, The Eating Disorders Program, The Hospital for Sick Children

Karin Jasper, PhD, MEd
Assistant Professor, Department of Psychiatry, University of Toronto Clinical Specialist, The Eating Disorders Day Hospital Program, The Hospital for Sick Children Associated Instructor, Department of Adult Education and Counselling Psychology, Ontario Institute for Studies in Education at University of Toronto

Natasha Johnson-Ramgeet, MD, FRCP(C)
Division of Adolescent Medicine, Department of Paediatrics, The Hospital for Sick Children and University of Toronto

Debra K. Katzman, MD, FRCP(C)
Associate Professor of Paediatrics, Head, Division of Adolescent Medicine, Department of Paediatrics, Medical Director, The Eating Disorders Program, The Hospital for Sick Children and University of Toronto

Nogah Kerem, MD
Fellow, Division of Adolescent Medicine Division, Department of Paediatrics and Department of Psychiatry, The Hospital for Sick Children

Karen Leslie, MD, FRCP (C)
Associate Professor of Paediatrics, Division of Adolescent Medicine, Department of Paediatrics, The Hospital for Sick Children and University of Toronto

Gail McVey, PhD, C Psych
Health Systems Research Scientist, Community Health Systems Resource Group, Director, Ontario Community Outreach Program for Eating

Disorders, Assistant Professor of Public Health Sciences, Faculty of Medicine, The Hospital for Sick Children and University of Toronto

Leora Pinhas, MD, FRCP(C)
Lecturer, Department of Psychiatry Psychiatric Director, The Eating Disorders Program The Hospital for Sick Children and University of Toronto

Gad Reisler, MD
Fellow, Division of Adolescent Medicine Division, Department of Paediatrics, The Hospital for Sick Children

Clare Roscoe, MD, FRCP(C)
Child Psychiatry, Fellow, Department of Psychiatry, The Hospital for Sick Children and University of Toronto

Donna Samuels, RN
Transition Planner/Community Liaison, The Eating Disorders Program, The Hospital for Sick Children

Patti Schabas, MD, FRCP(C)
Lecturer, Department of Psychiatry, The Eating Disorders Program, The Hospital for Sick Children and University of Toronto

Caitlin Shipley, MSW, RSW
The Eating Disorders Program, The Hospital for Sick Children

Kelly Sherwood, RD
Clinical Dietitian, The Eating Disorders Program, The Hospital for Sick Children

Tania Turrini, RD
Clinical Dietitian, The Eating Disorders Program, The Hospital for Sick Children

Kellie Welch, RD
Clinical Dietitian, The Eating Disorders Program, The Hospital for Sick Children

Blake Woodside, MD
Professor, Department of Psychiatry, Director, Inpatient Eating Disorder Program, The University Health Network and University of Toronto

Preface

As parents, we have great hopes that our children will grow and develop into healthy young adults without experiencing any difficulties along the way. However, some young people encounter problems with their eating attitudes and behaviors. Parents become confused and worried when their children experience weight loss, avoid food, become unhappy with the way they look, fear becoming 'fat', pick at their food, go on diets, exercise excessively, feel anxious about eating, isolate themselves from family and friends, and experience anxiety and depression that seems to be related to their eating behavior. Parents are right to be concerned about these behaviors. Eating disorders are the third most common chronic condition of adolescence. Eating disorders are life-threatening if not identified and treated at an early stage.

The experience of having a child or adolescent with an eating disorder can be extremely demanding and challenging for parents. This book is designed to provide parents with practical, commonsense information on these disorders, including how to identify the signs and symptoms of an eating disorder, what kinds of treatment are effective for eating disorders, and how families, friends, and other concerned community members can assist with your child's recovery. We also offer advice on how to ask your children if they have problems with eating; what to do if they have an eating problem but insist they don't; what to do if your children assure you that they can handle the eating disorder on their own; and how to cope with your frustrations and fear.

Help for Eating Disorders is written by an experienced interdisciplinary team of pediatric and adolescent medicine clinicians, including pediatricians, psychiatrists, dietitians, social workers, nurses, and psychologists. These experts combine the latest medical research with their extensive experience in treating children with eating disorders and counseling children and families.

The book is divided into three sections: diagnosis, treatment, and recovery. The first section focuses on understanding eating disorders, how they affect your child, and how best to determine if your child needs help. The second features information on the assessment and treatment of child and adolescent eating disorders. The third follows the course of recovery, focusing on what results to expect from treatment and how to manage your life and your child's life during this process.

Each chapter includes helpful case studies that bring to life specific eating disorder behaviors and attitudes. There are also two personal testimonials: one written by a parent of a young person who suffered from an eating disorder; and another by a young person who had anorexia nervosa as an adolescent and is now recovering. Many parents may see their own children mirrored in some way in these case studies and testimonials. They may gain courage from these personal accounts. These stories also remind us how emotionally challenging these disorders can be for parents and children.

Being a parent of a child with an eating disorder is a difficult job, but so is being a child or adolescent struggling with an eating disorder. We trust this book will provide you with practical information, support, and comfort as you and your child work through the process of diagnosis, treatment, and recovery.

PART 1

Diagnosing Eating Disorders

CHAPTER 1

What Is an Eating Disorder?

Eating disorders are illnesses that affect all aspects of a child's or adolescent's life. Eating disorders, such as anorexia nervosa, bulimia nervosa, and binge eating disorder, include extreme feelings, attitudes, and behaviors about weight and food issues. If a young person has intense concerns about body weight, shape, or size and is practicing excessive weight control behaviors, then that child or adolescent may have some form of an eating disorder. All eating disorders are serious problems that have emotional and physical problems associated with them. Children and adolescents can die from having an eating disorder.

EATING DISORDER FACTS

- Eating disorders are common among adolescents and young adults between the ages of 12 and 25 years old. Children as a young as 7 years old have been diagnosed with an eating disorder. The greatest risk is for girls between 14 and 18 years old.

- Eating disorder symptoms are very common. One in 8 adolescent girls have eating disorder symptoms that can be helped with treatment.

- Fewer than 1 in 10 adolescent girls with symptoms of an eating disorder seek an assessment for an eating disorder.

- Eating disorders are becoming more common in boys.

- At least 1 in 10 people who develop eating disorders are boys.

- Most children or adolescents get help for an eating disorder because their parents insist they get help...not because they want to get help.

- Children and adolescents with eating disorders need to seek professional help. The quicker an eating disorder is identified, the quicker they will get treatment and the better the outcome.

- Eating disorders can cause death.

What Is Anorexia Nervosa?

Anorexia nervosa is one type of eating disorder that is very difficult for many people to understand. Anorexia nervosa is a serious, potentially life-threatening disorder characterized by self-starvation and excessive weight loss. This disorder often begins during adolescence, frequently around the time of puberty. Anorexia nervosa affects about 1 in 100 adolescent girls. Anorexia nervosa is also found in boys.

Children and adolescents with anorexia nervosa have an overwhelming fear of being overweight and an extreme drive to be thin. This leads them to behaviors that will cause weight loss, including cutting back on what they eat in a way that can lead to being underweight. Children and adolescents with anorexia nervosa work hard to have strict control over their eating. The young person becomes obsessed with food and dieting. They may become dangerously thin. No matter how thin they get, they think they are still fat or they may be terrified about becoming fat.

Some young people will exercise a lot to burn off calories. They may count calories or fat grams, starve themselves, or limit the types of food they allow themselves to eat. They may attempt to get rid of the food they have eaten, purging themselves by self-induced vomiting or by taking laxatives. They may use diet pills to control appetite or take other medicines to control their weight. Family members may notice that the young person may deny hunger, make excuses to avoid eating, and avoid eating in front of anyone. They will often hide food they claim to have eaten.

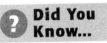

Did You Know...

● For every 10 girls who have anorexia nervosa, there will be one boy who has it.

● With treatment, about 75% to 80% of adolescents with an eating disorder will recover.

● Up to 20% of patients with eating disorders will eventually die of their illness.

What the Textbooks Say...

There is a textbook definition of anorexia nervosa that helps health-care professionals make a diagnosis. Anorexia nervosa is diagnosed based on specific characteristics or criteria. These criteria are most helpful for older adolescents and adults. Making a diagnosis of anorexia nervosa in a child or young adolescent is much more difficult. Evidence of any one of the following symptoms is cause for concern:

- Serious weight loss or failure to gain weight during a period of growth.
- Extreme fear of weight gain or becoming fat, even though the young person may be extremely underweight.

- Poor and distorted body image. People with anorexia nervosa are usually dissatisfied with their present weight, shape, and size. In addition, these young people cannot accurately see or understand their real body size. They often deny the seriousness of low body weight.
- In young girls who have had at least one menstrual period, the absence of at least three menstrual cycles in a row.

CASE STUDY Susan

When Susan decided to go on a diet, her father thought it was a good idea. He thought he should encourage her. After all, she would lose some of that baby fat. He also believed that this would be a good opportunity for her to practice some healthy eating behaviors. He told her that if she lost 10 pounds, she could buy a new outfit.

While she was dieting, he admired her willpower. Susan cut out all junk food and ate healthy. She went to the gym every day and did an intensive one-hour workout. When she lost the weight, he was proud of her achievement. You could always count on Susan succeeding once she set her mind to it. According to her father, Susan went from being a cute 13-year-old teenager to looking "like a model." He didn't suspect anything was wrong until she fainted at school one day.

When Susan fainted at school, she was immediately sent to the local emergency room. Her mother met her there. Both parents were shocked to find out that the doctor was admitting Susan to the hospital because she had a very slow heart rate and she was severely dehydrated. The doctor asked if Susan had lost any weight recently. Susan's mother was surprised to hear Susan proudly report that she had lost 35 pounds.

Had it really been that much? Both her parents were shocked and frightened. Seeing their daughter hooked up to a heart monitor was terrifying. How did this happen? They still had a hard time believing the slow heart rate was in some way related to her losing weight. Losing weight was supposed to improve your health, not have you end up in the hospital!

Over the next few days, her parents were stunned to hear that Susan was refusing to eat some of the food that was given to her and as a result was continuing to lose weight. This did not make sense. Their daughter had always been reasonable. If the doctor said that "good nutrition would help her heart," then why wasn't Susan eating? That's when they got the news. Susan had anorexia nervosa.

continued on page 26

What Is Bulimia Nervosa?

Bulimia nervosa is another type of eating disorder that often develops in the mid-teen years.

Bulimia nervosa often starts in a similar way to anorexia nervosa with an attempt to lose weight by eating less. Instead of continuing to starve themselves, young people with bulimia nervosa start to binge and purge.

Binging means that a young person eats a larger than normal amount of food in a relatively short period of time. Adolescents feel a lack of control over their eating behaviors when they are binging. After a binge, they purge. The need to purge is usually caused by fear of weight gain, stomach discomfort, or shame caused by the loss of control over eating.

Methods of purging may include vomiting, excessively exercising, fasting for a day or more after a binge, taking laxatives, diuretics, ipecac, or diet pills. The binging and purging is often done secretly. What makes bulimia nervosa different from anorexia nervosa is not the purging, but the cycle of binging and purging.

Young people with bulimia nervosa may be difficult to recognize because their weight may vary: they may be of average weight, above average weight, or below average weight. Family members may notice repeated episodes of rapid food consumption followed by tremendous guilt. They may also notice the young person regularly engaging in stringent diet plans and exercise.

There may be the misuse of laxatives, diuretics, or diet pills, a persistent concern with body image, making excuses to go to the bathroom immediately after meals, and eating large amounts of food without weight gain. There may be large and rapid fluctuations in weight as a result of chaotic eating behaviors. Children and adolescents with bulimia nervosa may be caught throwing up in the bathroom or there may be evidence of vomiting.

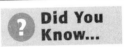

Did You Know...

● Bulimia nervosa is thought to occur in 5 out of every 100 women.

● We know less about the long-term outcome, but likely 5% to 10% may die from the illness.

What the Textbooks Say...

There is a textbook definition of bulimia nervosa that helps health-care professionals make a diagnosis. These features are generally accepted as being characteristic of bulimia nervosa. As with anorexia nervosa, evidence of any one of the following characteristics in a child or adolescent is cause for concern:

- Repeated episodes of binging where an unusually large amount of food is eaten in a short period of time (2 hours) and the person feels out of control.
- Repeated attempts to compensate for the binges in ways that are often unhealthy, such as vomiting, using laxatives, or exercising excessively.
- Episodes of binging and then compensating occur twice a week for 3 months.
- Young people's sense of self is greatly affected by their perception of their weight or shape.

CASE STUDY Martha

Martha had always been a determined child; she had to be, being the youngest with three older brothers around. At 16 years old, her mother was worried that she was getting a little "wild." Martha was hanging out with a group of kids her parents didn't approve of, she was missing curfews, and her grades at school were starting to slip. What next?

Her mother's real concern was with the new behavior Martha had developed. Just before a meal was over, she would excuse herself from the table to go to the bathroom. She would spend 20 to 30 minutes there.

The family would hear the water running for long periods of time. Her brothers gave her a hard time as it appeared that Martha had found the perfect way to avoid cleaning up after meals.

Martha's parents were very concerned that she was spending too much time in the bathroom. They were worried that she was throwing up. Her parents started lingering outside the bathroom door listening for evidence. Martha gave it to them. Despite the sound of the running water, her father heard her throwing up and her mother clearly caught an odor of vomit in the bathroom.

continued on page 22

What Is Binge Eating Disorder?

Binge eating disorder is a relatively newly recognized eating disorder in children and adolescents. It is characterized by eating an unusually large amount of food, eating until one is uncomfortable, eating quickly and secretly during the binge episodes, and feeling guilty, ashamed, or depressed after binge eating. This disorder in children and younger adolescents is associated with eating when the young person is not hungry.

Young people with binge eating disorder use eating to try to change uncomfortable emotional feelings, such as feeling angry, sad, bored, or worried. They often eat in secret or hide food. Many young people with this problem are either above average weight or obese, but normal-weight adolescents can have the disorder. Unlike adults, dieting is not a major factor in the binge eating disorder found in children and younger adolescents. Some young people who develop binge eating disorder may struggle with depression.

What the Textbooks Say...

The textbook definition of binge eating disorder is so new it is still undergoing changes. As with anorexia nervosa or bulimia nervosa, evidence of any one of the following symptoms is cause for concern:

- Recurrent episodes of binge eating. An episode of binge eating is characterized by both of the following:
  - Food seeking in the absence of hunger (e.g., after a full meal).
  - A sense of lack of control over eating (e.g., "When I start to eat, I just can't stop").
- Binge episodes are associated with one or more of the following:
  - Food seeking in response to negative affect (e.g., sadness, boredom, restlessness).
  - Food seeking as a reward.
  - Sneaking or hiding food.
- Symptoms persist over a period of 3 months.
- Eating is not associated with the regular use of inappropriate compensatory behaviors (e.g., purging, fasting, excessive exercise) and does not occur exclusively during the course of anorexia nervosa or bulimia nervosa.

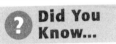

Did You Know...

- Binge eating disorder is different from bulimia nervosa. After they binge eat, adolescents with bulimia nervosa will purge by vomiting, using diuretics ('water' pills) or laxatives, fasting, or doing excessive exercise to keep from gaining weight. Adolescents with binge eating disorder may not purge.

CASE STUDY Jessica

My out-of-control eating started when I was 14 years old. I was a bit overweight. At least that was what everyone in my immediate family would tell me. My family members were always critical of my body weight and size. It would not be uncommon to hear my older brother say, "You could stand to lose a few pounds," or my mother to say, "I'm not sure I'd eat that cookie…you want to get into that new dress we just bought!"

I really wanted to lose some weight. So, I followed a bunch of different diets that I found in teen magazines. Yes, I tried them all. But nothing seemed to work. I think I tried about 15 to 20 different diets over the span of 4 months. Instead of losing weight, I started to gain weight. After a day of dieting, I was terribly hungry. I would often go to the kitchen late at night and eat anything and everything I could get my hands on. I was very secretive about it. I would eat and eat and eat…until I was beyond full.

I would feel horrible afterward…guilty, angry, hateful. I would hate myself for doing this. This didn't just happen once…it happened three to four times a week. I hate it.

continued on page 49

Eating Disorder Not Otherwise Specified

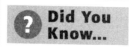

Did You Know…

• Young people in the category of Eating Disorders Not Otherwise Specified still have a serious condition that can be life threatening.

Many children and adolescents who have eating disorders may not have all the characteristics that fit into anorexia nervosa, bulimia nervosa, or binge eating disorder. They may have one or more but not all of the symptoms. Young people who are just developing these disorders and have not had them for a long period of time may not have all the characteristics of these disorders. For these children and adolescents, there is another eating disorder category called Eating Disorders Not Otherwise Specified (EDNOS).

Children and adolescents who fall into the category of Eating Disorder Not Otherwise Specified can have any combination of the characteristics that don't fit into anorexia nervosa, bulimia nervosa, or binge eating disorder.

CASE STUDY Brad

Brad had always been a worrier and a germ freak. Even when he was a little boy, he had to have things "just so." When he was 5 years old, he watched a television program on pollution and began having nightmares about it. What kid worries so much about pollution?

Brad was excited about going to school until the day he started kindergarten. Then he didn't want to go to school. He would beg his parents not to leave him at school. He would scream and cry. It would not stop until his parents agreed to stay with him in class.

The teacher called it "school refusal" and suggested that Brad and his parents get some help from a counselor. His parents were devastated and blamed themselves for Brad's behavior. They just assumed that it had something to do with their recent divorce.

Brad and his family met with a therapist who worked with them in an effort to return Brad to school immediately. Things settled down. Four years later, Brad's mother was planning on getting married. Brad was now 9 years old and doing well in school, had lots of friends, and seemed generally happy. Brad really liked his mom's fiancé and was very excited about the upcoming marriage.

Two months after the wedding, Brad got food poisoning. He couldn't stop throwing-up for a week. He lost about 5 pounds, which was a lot for someone of his body size. Thereafter, he became afraid to eat almost anything that could go "bad." It was becoming a real challenge making his lunches and dinners — everything had to come from a sealed container or be cooked so long it lost its flavor. Even then, he was unlikely to finish his meal.

Brad's parents were having a difficult time coping with this behavior. They were getting very impatient with his eating and unreasonable demands around food preparation. Brad's mother was worried about his health and began to feel increasingly inadequate when he would reject the food she made. Brad's parents talked about going to see their pediatrician for some help and advice.

continued on page 28

When Should You Worry?

Parents frequently ask two questions: "How do I know if my child has an eating disorder" and "How will I recognize whether my child has an eating disorder?" These are not easy questions to answer. Eating disorders are complicated to understand and can be a challenge to recognize. Many teenagers successfully hide these serious and sometimes fatal disorders from their families for many months or years.

You may have to deal with tears, tantrums, denials, or promises to do better. Don't let this interfere with your responsibility to get your child the care needed. Remember, young people die from these disorders.

WORKSHEET

GENERAL SYMPTOMS OF EATING DISORDERS

Here are some factors you should look for if you suspect that your child or adolescent has an eating disorder. Check off any signs that apply to your child and consult with your doctor if you have any concerns.

☐ Recent unexplained weight loss

☐ Fear of gaining weight or of being overweight

☐ Distorted image of their body's weight, shape, or size (for example, believing that they are overweight even though they are at a healthy weight or underweight)

☐ No or little growth in height at an age when children or adolescents should be growing

☐ No or little weight gain or weight loss at a time when there should be weight gain

☐ Significant fluctuation in weight

☐ Hoarding or hiding food

☐ Purging behaviors (vomiting, using diuretics or laxatives, or excessively exercising to lose weight)

☐ Preoccupation with thoughts of food, calories, exercise, and their weight

☐ Skipping meals, fasting, or eliminating entire food groups (restrictive eating patterns)

☐ Counting calories or grams of fat in food

☐ Preferring to eat alone

☐ Amenorrhea (absence of menstrual cycles) or delayed onset of puberty and menarche (a girl's first menstrual period)

☐ Exercising compulsively

☐ Extreme denial that they may have an eating disorder

☐ Withdrawing from friends and family

☐ Wearing baggy or layered clothing to hide weight loss or to keep warm

☐ Continual weight-checking and examining themselves in the mirror

☐ Reading food-related magazines, cookbooks, recipes, watching cooking shows on TV

☐ Enjoying discussing dieting issues

☐ Cooking and baking for others but rarely eating the baked and cooked food themselves

WORKSHEET

RELATED SYMPTOMS

Some young people with eating disorders may also have some struggles that are not related to the eating disorder but tend to show up in the same person.

☐ They may struggle with depression, anxiety or obsessive behaviors not related to food.

☐ They may be impulsive.

☐ They may participate in risky behaviors that can endanger them.

☐ They may want to or have a history of hurting themselves or have suicidal thoughts.

Communication Strategies

If you suspect that your daughter or son may be struggling with an eating disorder, the first thing to do is to speak with them. It can be helpful to describe what you have noticed and how it makes you feel. Let your children know that you are worried about their health and well-being. Try something like this:

- "I've noticed that you're losing a lot of weight. I'm worried that there may be something wrong with your health."
- "I've noticed that you're very critical about your body weight and shape. I'm worried that this is a problem for you."
- "I'm concerned that the way you are feeling is affecting how you are eating. I'm worried that this is a problem for you."
- "I've noticed that you are going to the bathroom right after every meal and spending a long time in there. I can't help thinking that something is wrong. Can we talk about it?"

If your child denies any problems, trust your instinct. If you have even the slightest intuition that there is something wrong, take your child to your doctor as soon as possible. This can be difficult and scary for you and your child. It is not uncommon for young people with an eating disorder to downplay the seriousness of their illness. Your child may not be completely honest about what is going on. Therefore, it is important for you to go with your child to provide additional information and inform the doctor about your concerns.

CHAPTER 2

What Are the Myths and Misconceptions about Eating Disorders?

Although progress has been made in the identification and treatment of children and adolescents with eating disorders, many myths and misconceptions about these disorders persist. Dispelling these myths is not only valuable for understanding the true nature of eating disorders, but also for removing the stigma often attached to children with these disorders. Since anorexia nervosa was first named as an eating disorder almost simultaneously by two doctors, Charles Lasegue (1873) in France and Sir William Gull (1874) in England, it has presented many challenges to medical science. Many people still struggle to accept it as a valid illness, and even when it is accepted, there are still controversies about how to help people, especially adolescents, struggling with it.

Myths and misconceptions about illness and healing have been with us for hundreds of years. This is especially true for mental illnesses, including eating disorders. Many misconceptions remain unchallenged in the collective mind. These misconceptions become a fertile ground for the creation of myths that reinforce misunderstanding and can have deleterious results.

Eating disorders are no exception. Myths and misconceptions often delay the ability of parents and health-care professionals to identify the problems and begin appropriate treatment. Such unnecessary delays have led to poorer outcomes with these difficult, but treatable, illnesses.

> **? Did You Know...**
>
> • Dispelling these myths is very important in the diagnosis, treatment, and recovery of children and adolescents with eating disorders.

EATING DISORDERS QUIZ

Mark with a "T" the statements you think are true, and with an "F" the statements you think are false. Answers are given at the end of the quiz and explanations follow in the rest of the chapter.

1. Adolescents with eating disorders come from dysfunctional families.

2. All fat adolescents are unhealthy.

3. You can never fully recover from an eating disorder.

4. You must know why you have an eating disorder to recover.

5. With a sensible diet and a strong commitment, everyone can become and remain thin.

6. Parents are part of the solution to an eating disorder.

7. You can always tell if people are anorexic by their appearance.

8. You are only bulimic if you eat a huge amount and then throw up afterward.

9. Anorexics do not eat candy, chocolate, or chips.

10. Compulsive eating, or binge eating, is not an eating disorder.

11. You cannot die from bulimia.

12. If you can get a person with anorexia to eat, that will solve the problem.

13. The only person needing support is the person with the eating disorder.

14. Only white teenage girls from well-to-do families get eating disorders.

15. If you eat three meals a day and don't purge, you don't have an eating disorder.

Answers: 1. F, 2. F, 3. F, 4. F, 5. F, 6. T, 7. F, 8. F, 9. F, 10. F, 11. F, 12. F, 13. F, 14. F, 15. F

What Is…and Is Not an Eating Disorder?

Eating disorders are only a problem with food…

No. Eating disorders are symptoms of underlying problems. Food and weight control are used as a tool to manage or solve problems that may seem otherwise impossible to solve. Both food restriction and binging can help some adolescents block out or numb painful feelings and emotions temporarily. For others, food can be used as comfort.

CASE STUDY Martha

Martha's parents sat her down one evening to discuss what they were observing. Martha rolled her eyes. She hated these talks. Her dad asked, "Why are you going to the bathroom immediately after you eat?" Martha became defensive and replied, "What do you think people do in the bathroom?" With great trepidation, Martha's mother replied, "I think you're throwing up!" It felt good to say that. Martha got angry. They argued. Martha's parents insisted that she be honest with them. They expressed how concerned they were about her vomiting and insisted she stop this behavior immediately. Martha denied that she was vomiting and told them, "Mind your own business!"

After the discussion, Martha stopped going to the bathroom after meals. Her mother or father would only occasionally find her spending an excessive amount of time in the bathroom. Still, her parents were on guard and vigilant about Martha's every move. They continued to argue about the amount of time she spent in the bathroom. "Anyone would think that it was not okay to 'pee' in this house," Martha would yell.

One evening, in an attempt to make peace and reconnect, Martha's mother was helping her with the laundry. She opened Martha's drawer and found a stash of laxatives. Martha tried to insist that they weren't hers. Then she tried to convince her mother that they were old and she hadn't used them in months. Martha's mother was shocked, frightened, and speechless.

Finally, Martha's mother sat her down and acknowledged that she was afraid of Martha's behavior and was really concerned that something was wrong. "I want you to see Dr. Brown as soon as I can get an appointment," she said. "There really is no choice in this matter. Your dad and I are concerned about your health and well-being. We all need some help! You need some help!" Martha reluctantly agreed.

continued on page 43

You can always tell if people have an eating disorder by their appearance...

Not everyone who has anorexia nervosa appears underweight. Not everyone with bulimia nervosa is slender. Not everyone who compulsively eats is large. Because there is a range of naturally occurring body sizes and shapes, the effect of an eating disorder on an adolescent's appearance varies with their background. Eating disorders are serious mental and physical health problems that are not only dependent on size or shape. It is also important to remember that not every adolescent who is really thin has an eating disorder.

Adolescents with anorexia nervosa do not eat candy, chocolate, or chips...

Anorexia nervosa is not about the *type* of food adolescents eat, but about the total amount of food they allow themselves in one day (along with how they balance this with the energy they use).

Adolescents with anorexia nervosa do not binge or purge, while those with bulimia nervosa do not restrict...

In fact, some adolescents with anorexia nervosa do have binges followed by purging behavior, and some adolescents purge even when they do not binge. Teens with bulimia nervosa most often restrict their food intake, which is often what leads to their binging.

If you eat three meals a day and never purge, you cannot have an eating disorder...

While eating three meals a day may seem to be a non-disordered eating pattern, it is disordered eating if the food choices are intended to keep the person from maintaining a healthy weight.

You only have bulimia nervosa if you eat a huge amount and then throw up or use laxatives afterward...

Eating a large amount of food in a short period of time and experiencing this behavior as being out of control is part of bulimia nervosa. Adolescents with bulimia nervosa compensate for this large amount of food intake by purging. Purging

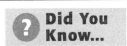
Did You Know...

● Although adolescents do not have more than one eating disorder at a time, it is not unusual for them to have different eating disorders at different times.

● Approximately 30% of teenagers with anorexia nervosa will develop bulimia nervosa.

● What's important is not so much what type of disorder a person has, but rather the impact of the illness on the individual.

behaviors, such as vomiting and using laxatives, are not the only ways adolescents get rid of food they ate. Exercise, fasting, and restricting food intake are a few examples that may also be considered purging behaviors.

If you are above/on the high end of your healthy weight range, you cannot possibly have an eating disorder...

In the case of anorexia nervosa, being at a healthy weight is one part of recovery, but another part is attending to the emotional and psychological issues that accompanied the weight loss. With bulimia nervosa, even during the active stages, weight is usually within the healthy range. Recovery may not mean a big change in weight, but does require dealing with the binging and purging, as well as the emotional, psychological, and physical issues that accompany these behaviors.

What Are Common Myths about Eating Disorders?

Boys with eating disorders are always gay...

This is false. Some research has suggested that boys who are homosexual have a higher risk of developing an eating disorder than boys who are not. However, both anorexia nervosa and bulimia nervosa affect straight boys as well.

Barbie and Ken represent ideal body shapes for females and males...

The body shapes of these doll figures are in fact impossible to attain for real human beings. If Barbie were a real woman, her proportions would cause her to fall over. Ken would be 7 feet, 8 inches tall. His neck would be 8 inches bigger than the average male's. Ken and other male action figures, like G.I. Joe, are now being made much bigger and more muscular than they were 20 years ago. The female models we see in fashion magazines do not represent any meaningful ideal for the majority of females. In fact, only 1 in 10,000 females naturally (without dieting) meet model-thin dimensions.

All fat adolescents are unhealthy...

Being 'fat' means different things to different people. Sometimes kids will refer to others as fat because they look a certain way or because they want to be hurtful. Remember that there is a wide range of healthy weights in children and adolescents. In fact, many adolescents who would be seen as fat by today's cultural standards are completely healthy. Being at the extreme ends of the weight range — for instance, being too thin or extremely obese — can be associated with health risks. If you have concerns about your child's health, you should check with your doctor. Everyone, regardless of weight, shape, or size should focus on healthy living, which means eating a nutritious diet and exercising moderately.

To be thin is to be happy...

Our culture associates positive qualities with thinness and negative qualities with fatness. Media personalities and advertising reinforce the idea that being thin brings with it all of the rewards our culture values: success, love, and happiness. If this were really true, teenagers with eating disorders would all be happy. However, as most teens struggling with an eating disorder will tell you, weight loss does not automatically bring happiness. We all know adolescents of different sizes and shapes with different life circumstances who are happy.

With a sensible diet and a strong commitment, everyone can become and remain thin...

Research suggests that our weight and shape are largely affected by our genetic makeup. Nutrition and exercise can influence weight and shape to a degree, just as nutrition can affect height, but overall weight and height are determined by genetics. Not everyone can be 6-feet tall and not everyone can be thin. Recent research studies confirm that, over the long term, dieting tends to result in increased weight rather than decreased weight.

You have to exercise a lot for it to do any good...

Actually, a person can do too much exercise — overexercising can be harmful. Exercise can be good for one's health, if done in moderation. Current research suggests that accumulating 150 minutes of moderate activity a week provides significant health benefits.

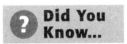

Did You Know...

• Eating disorders were once thought to affect only white adolescent girls from well-to-do families. Research studies have shown that this is in fact false.

• Eating disorders affect males as well as females.

• A person with an eating disorder may be from any racial, ethnic, or economic background; and a person may be of any age and any sexual orientation.

CASE STUDY Susan

Susan was admitted to her local hospital for a few days after fainting at school. The doctors felt it was due to her weight loss. They suggested moving her to another hospital, where they had a special unit to treat children and adolescents with eating problems. At first, Susan's parents were reluctant to move their daughter to an eating disorder unit – their daughter couldn't have an eating disorder! However, the doctor convinced them it was a good idea for the other team to do a thorough inpatient assessment. Susan's parents agreed. They were certain that the eating disorder experts would find another medical reason for their daughter's weight loss. Surely, she was losing weight for some other reason!

Three days later, Susan was transferred and admitted to the eating disorder ward. Within a couple of days, Susan was complaining that she hated it there . . . so many rules and everyone treated her like she was "sick." Susan didn't feel sick. Her parents could see that she was distressed being in the hospital. Susan tried to convince her parents that she was not like the other kids on the ward.

"I don't have an eating disorder…I have no problem gaining weight and getting better!" Susan went about proving it, too. She followed all the rules and started gaining weight. Susan's father was relieved – this was his daughter, setting her mind to something and succeeding.

The treatment team was cautious with both Susan and her parents. It's not unusual for adolescents with eating disorders to follow the rules while they are in hospital. One of the doctors informed Susan's parents that kids manage to gain weight initially, particularly when they are acutely medically unwell. However, as they gain weight, it often gets harder to keep going. But Susan's father thought, 'They don't know my daughter!'

continued on page 34

Why Do Adolescents Develop Eating Disorders?

People with eating disorders come from dysfunctional families…

The causes of eating disorders are unknown. Teens from a full range of family types can develop eating disorders, so we know that it is not the family that causes them. It was once thought that autism was caused by parents who were detached and uncaring. In other words, parents were blamed if their child was autistic. Later, it was discovered that autism is a neurologic disorder.

Sometimes the difficulties of having someone in your family with an eating disorder may make it appear as if your family is dysfunctional. Health-care professionals can help a family identify any patterns that may contribute to the continuation of the eating disorder and provide them with strategies that will assist in the recovery process. Parents should be viewed as part of the solution, not the cause of the problem.

Adolescents with eating disorders do this to hurt their family and friends...

Seeing the effects of an eating disorder on a loved one is very painful. However, adolescents with eating disorders do not usually intend to cause pain to their family and friends. Typically, they tend to protect family members from knowing what they are going through. This is part of the secretiveness of the illness.

Bulimia nervosa is a good way to lose weight — to have your cake and eat it too...

Bulimia nervosa is an illness, with serious medical and psychological consequences, including the possibility of death. It is not an effective or safe way to lose weight.

Adolescents who binge or eat compulsively are just lazy...

Binge eating is a disordered eating pattern, just like anorexia and bulimia nervosa. All three eating patterns use food to cope with difficult emotions and circumstances. They express emotional pain. Adolescents who binge eat are not lazy; they need proper treatment. Diets and spas are not forms of treatment.

? Did You Know...

• An eating disorder is not just a phase of growing up, nor a phase of dieting. It is a real medical disorder that most often requires professional help.

• Assuming that an eating disorder will go away on its own can contribute to the severity of the disorder.

What Can You Do?

The only person needing support is the adolescent with the eating disorder...

While support for the adolescent with the eating disorder is very important, family members and friends need support, too. Eating disorders are potentially long term or chronic illnesses. Supporting the caregivers and siblings improves the possibility of recovery. Professional guidance also helps the parents and siblings to cope with the illness.

You can rely on your doctor's opinion...

Eating disorders are not always identified by an adolescent's appearance. A good medical and psychosocial history, as well as a complete physical examination by a doctor, will usually make it easier for the complicated symptoms of an eating disorder to be recognized. However, adolescents with eating disorders tend to be more aware of their own symptoms and may not tell the doctors what they need to know. Not all medical schools provide training in eating disorders. If you are in doubt, seek a second opinion.

If I just get her to eat it, that will solve the problem... If I can keep him out of the bathroom, that will solve the problem...

While helping children or adolescents suffering from an eating disorder deal with their physical symptoms is important for recovery, there are other aspects of the eating disorder, including feeling and thinking patterns, that need to be addressed for full recovery. Otherwise, an adolescent who has anorexia nervosa, for instance, may eat because she feels she has no choice or is being supported to eat, but may find a way of getting around this, for example, by overexercising.

CASE STUDY Brad

Brad's biologic parents decided he needed help. All three of them sat down for a serious discussion. During the divorce, his parents decided that they would not bring him into their issues. When it came to issues concerning Brad, they would work as a parental unit with his best interests in mind. The only way this would work is if they stuck to the ground rules they learned when they went to mediation during the divorce. They stuck to "I feel" statements.

Brad's mother started. She told him that when she watched him struggle so much with his eating, she became worried about him. She was worried that he would get sick if he did not eat more. His father told him that it was hard to see him worry so much about eating, and it was upsetting that he could not enjoy his favorite foods anymore. His stepfather told him that he wanted to help, but did not know how, and that this made him sad. His parents told him it was time to go to the therapist again.

Brad agreed reluctantly. Brad wasn't sure it would help, but his parents were worried and they usually decided when it was time to see the doctor. It helped last time.

continued on page 44

You cannot die from an eating disorder...

Eating disorders have one of the highest death rates of any psychiatric disorder. While the death rate among adolescents suffering with eating disorders is usually estimated to be 5% to 9%, some researchers have reported rates of up to 20% in chronically ill adults. Adolescents with bulimia nervosa are equally vulnerable as those with anorexia nervosa.

Can Anyone Ever Recover?

When an adolescent enters a treatment program, the problem goes away quickly...

Treatment programs do not make eating disorders go away. They usually are the initial stage of recovery, and even then, they depend on the way the adolescent makes use of them. To assume that an adolescent with an eating disorder will get well shortly after entering a treatment program will put undue pressure on them and may interfere with the recovery process. Recovery typically takes up to 5 years or longer.

There is a deep underlying issue that must be uncovered before getting well ... Someone must know why they have an eating disorder in order to recover...

The causes of eating disorders are not known. Many factors may contribute to the development of eating disorders, including underlying issues. However, once the eating disorder is established, resolving these underlying issues will not necessarily resolve the eating disorder.

Recovering from an eating disorder is just like recovering from alcoholism...

While eating disorders and alcoholism can both be coping mechanisms, there are important differences when it comes to the recovery process. One path to recovery from alcoholism is to stop drinking altogether, but recovery from an eating disorder cannot happen through the avoidance of food or particular types of food. It requires learning to eat a full range of foods without compensating for eating by exercising or other behaviors.

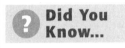

Did You Know...

• Children and adolescents can fully recover from all types of eating disorders. According to research studies, the majority of adolescents with eating disorders do recover.

• The outcome is better for young people with eating disorders who get treatment early on.

CHAPTER 3

Who Is at Risk for Developing an Eating Disorder?

Any child or adolescent can develop an eating disorder, but there are some young people who are at higher risk. A risk factor is something that increases the chances of getting a disorder but is not a direct cause of the disorder. A number of risk factors can play a role in your child's risk of developing an eating disorder. Not all children and adolescents who develop an eating disorder have risk factors. However, the more risk factors your child has, the greater the chances of your child developing an eating disorder.

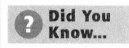 **Did You Know...**

• Eating disorders are more common among adolescents and young adults.

• Eating disorders commonly develop between the ages of 12 and 25 years old.

• The period of greatest risk for girls is between the ages of 14 and 18.

Gender

In general, girls are more likely than boys to develop eating disorders. About 90% of adolescents with eating disorders are females. Recent research has shown that eating disorders are more widespread in males than previously thought. In fact, 1 in 5 adolescents with anorexia nervosa under 14 years old are boys.

Socioeconomic Class

Children and adolescents from all social and economic classes living in an economically developed country are at risk for developing an eating disorder. In economically developed countries, bulimia nervosa may be higher among lower socioeconomic groups.

Ethnicity

Eating disorders are becoming more common around the world. Eating disorders occur in children and adolescents from almost every culture and ethnic group. No one is spared.

Dieting

Research studies have shown that there is a link between dieting and the development of eating disorders in teenagers. It is not uncommon for adolescents to feel unhappy about their body weight, shape, and size at some time. One study showed that 78% of teenaged girls would like to weigh less. Some adolescents can become preoccupied with food and fat, frequently ending up on a diet. In fact, it is rare to find a teen who, by the age of 18, has not yet experimented with dieting.

Adolescent girls who diet are more likely to develop an eating disorder than girls who do not diet. Not every dieter will develop an eating disorder, but nearly every eating disorder begins with some kind of attempt at weight loss.

> **? Did You Know...**
>
> • Approximately, 80% of teen girls and 10% of teen boys have been on a diet by age 13.
>
> • About 1 in 3 young people who diet will progress to serious dieting, and 25% of these serious dieters will develop abnormal eating attitudes and behaviors or an eating disorder.

Childhood Obesity

Childhood obesity is one of the risk factors for the development of an eating disorder. Overweight children tend to show a greater concern with weight, shape, and eating, as well as a greater tendency to dietary restraint.

Low Self-Esteem and Depression

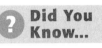

Low self-esteem and symptoms of depression are associated with childhood obesity. Both of these may also increase the risk of developing an eating disorder.

Genetic Predisposition

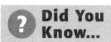

Recent research has shown that genes may contribute to the onset of an eating disorder. Genes are sections of DNA that are carried on chromosomes and that determine specific human characteristics, such as height or eye color. Some characteristics come from a single gene, whereas others come from a number of genes acting together. One gene is not likely responsible for anorexia nervosa or bulimia nervosa. More likely, a number of genes contribute to a person's vulnerability to develop an eating disorder. This does not mean that emotional, behavioral, and environmental reasons do not play an important role in the development of an eating disorder.

Personality Traits

Anorexia nervosa is more common in children and adolescents who are perfectionists, have low self-esteem, and do not like the way their body's look. Some adolescents at risk

HELP FOR DISCUSSING RISK FACTORS WITH YOUR CHILD

Here are a few tips for parents if they are concerned that their child has risk factors associated with the development of an eating disorder. Parents should approach their child with their concerns. Parents should also seek advice from their child's doctor.

• Do not hesitate to approach your child with your concerns about their eating attitudes and behaviors.

• Encourage open dialog. Talk to your daughter or son if you are concerned about their attitudes and behaviors.

• Promote free expression of thoughts and feelings.

• Be sensitive and nonjudgmental.

• Listen with no interruptions.

• Be attentive to all the changes in your children's lives as they grow and develop.

• Observe and monitor your child's home and school life, including academic progress, social life, and extracurricular activities.

• Seek professional help. Visit a health-care professional who is knowledgeable about the health and well-being of children and adolescents.

for developing anorexia nervosa have fears about growing up and becoming independent adults. Adolescents with anorexia nervosa are often rigid in their thinking. For example, they evaluate their thoughts and situations into extremes, such as 'black or white,' 'good or bad,' and 'fat or thin.'

Adolescents with eating disorders have difficulty with change — changes in their daily activity and social situations, changes in their body. Adolescents with bulimia nervosa have problems with impulse control. This means they often act or speak without considering the consequences. Adolescents with anorexia nervosa, bulimia nervosa or binge eating disorders handle stress, pressure, and nervousness through abnormal eating behaviors.

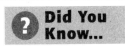

Early Puberty

There seems to be a greater risk for the development of eating disorders in girls who experience early puberty. Puberty is a time when numerous changes occur, including the development of body image concerns, shape preoccupation, body dissatisfaction, and dieting. Puberty is also a time when physical changes occur, including a normal increase in body fat in girls. If a normal increase in body fat occurs while your daughter's peers still have childish body shapes, this can lead to feelings of being too fat. Being one of the first in a group of teens to go through puberty can cause teasing and unwanted attention. This may result in an attempt to restrict food intake and lose weight.

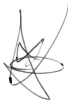

? Did You Know...

• Girls who are nutritionally deprived because of restricting their diet can slow down or stop their pubertal development.

Sexual Orientation

There is limited research on connections between eating disorders and sexual orientation. To date, nothing indicates that an adolescent's sexual preference influences the development of an eating disorder.

Competitive Athletics

Adolescents who participate in highly competitive athletic activities, where body weight, shape, and size are emphasized, show a greater risk of developing an eating disorder. Girls participating in gymnastics, figure skating, ballet, track, and cross-country running are at particular risk for eating disorders. Boys who are wrestlers or lightweight rowers are also at risk for manipulating their weight and developing disordered eating behaviors.

CASE STUDY Susan

Over the next few weeks, Susan slowly gained weight. The team thought she was well enough to go on a weekend pass home. The family was very excited. As Susan's parents expected, the pass went well and Susan even gained a little weight. Susan's parents really felt reassured that she did not have an eating disorder…her weight loss was just a phase she was going through. Once she was out, things would go back to normal. Susan agreed. Now that she had one successful pass home, she started to ask her parents to sign her out of the hospital. After all, she had proven she could gain even at home. Her mother was a bit nervous about taking her home. Susan's mother thought about what life was like just before her daughter's admission to the hospital. Why was Susan able to gain weight in the hospital but lost all that weight before she came into the hospital?

Susan was relentless with her parents… she wanted to go home! She missed her friends, was falling behind in school, and was doing everything her parents had asked her to do…even gaining weight! She could clearly do this at home. Her parents asked the treatment team if she could come home.

The team was reluctant. They felt that while Susan had gained some weight, she still remained underweight. They were concerned about Susan's ability to continue her weight gain at home. This was particularly important as she was in the midst of her adolescent growth and development. The treatment team also expressed concern that Susan had not been participating well in the psychological part of the admission.

Susan's parents were confused. They felt their daughter was fine. They were clear that she was going to continue to gain the weight outside of the hospital. They were also hesitant about their daughter participating in the group sessions on the ward…these sessions did not seem appropriate for an adolescent who didn't have an eating disorder. Their daughter was not like the other kids.

continued on page 39

Occupations

There is a higher risk of eating disorders among models and actors, who may experience social and professional pressures to be thin.

Bullying

Bullying is an aggressive behavior that occurs repeatedly over time, is intended to cause harm, and involves an imbalance of power between the child who bullies and the child who is bullied. Among boys, bullying typically involves pushing, shoving, and other forms of physical intimidation. Girls tend to bully through gossiping, social exclusion, and verbal teasing. Kids involved in this torment can have lasting social and emotional problems.

Bullying can negatively affect your child's self-esteem and self-confidence. It can be particularly concerning if the bullying relates to the young person's weight or body size. Children learn very early in life that "fat" is a bad word and will use it when calling each other names.

Chronic Illness (Diabetes)

Eating disorders are particularly dangerous for young people with diabetes. Having both can be life threatening and cause long-term complications.

Diabetes can create a preoccupation with food. It can also result in the need for parents to take control over the young person's life. These factors, as well as the increased weight gain that insulin treatment can cause, may contribute to the increased risk associated with eating disorders.

In addition, low blood glucose or hypoglycemia can occur in a young person who restricts food intake or purges. High blood glucose or hyperglycemia can occur because of binge eating. Hyperglycemia can be so severe as to cause ketoacidosis (a serious medical condition requiring immediate medical treatment that occurs when the body uses fat as an energy source and ketones build up in the blood). This condition can lead to death.

? Did You Know...

- Low-self esteem is a risk factor for the development of an eating disorder.

- According to one survey, 10 out of 100 teenage girls and 7 out of 100 teenage boys with chronic illness, such as diabetes or asthma, have an eating disorder.

Social and Cultural Pressures

Teenagers in Western culture are under pressure to be thin. Our society is filled with unrealistic images of young people. Images of thin, beautiful, successful people are constantly portrayed in the media. Magazines are filled with images of wasted models. Television shows portray underweight actors. Television, computers, and magazine advertisements are filled with diet commercials, weight-loss products, and the newest exercise regimens. The message from our appearance-obsessed society is clear: to be happy is to be thin! Along with other pressures, social and cultural images of the body can lead to higher rates of eating disorders in teens.

> **? Did You Know...**
>
> • Approximately 50% to 60% of children and adolescents with eating disorders experience depression or anxiety.

Psychiatric Disorders

Children and adolescents with depression, obsessive-compulsive, and anxiety disorders are at greater risk for developing an eating disorder. Depression is a treatable mental illness that can have emotional and physical effects, such as feelings of sadness, worthlessness, guilt, and indecision. It can lead to difficulty in concentrating; change in appetite or sleep habits; and loss of energy, interest, or pleasure. Anxiety disorders involve intense anxiety and cause distress.

Physical and Sexual Abuse

Adolescents who have been abused describe using the eating disorder as a way of coping with the painful feelings and memories. Children and adolescents have described using vomiting as a means of cleansing themselves or as a way of punishing themselves for being 'bad' and not deserving to be nurtured. Young people with a history of abuse almost always need professional help to find healthier ways to cope.

However, research suggests that children and adolescents who have been sexually abused have about the same or only a slightly higher incidence of eating disorders as those who have not been mistreated. Abused children and adolescents are more likely to have mental health issues than those who have not been abused.

WORKSHEET

LIFE EVENTS AFFECTING EATING DISORDERS

Listed here are experiences that young people with eating disorders have identified as having influenced their eating behavior. Check "Yes" if you believe the experience has influenced your child's eating disorder, "No" if not. If in doubt, check the "Don't Know" box. After completing this checklist, you may want to discuss the "Yes" and "Don't Know" responses with your child and your doctor.

Life Event	Yes	No	Don't Know
Interpersonal Concerns			
Bullying or teasing in general or specifically about weight, body shape, and physical appearance.	☑	☐	☐
Friends focusing on dieting and body image.	☑	☐	☐
Participating in a weight-related activity at school or in a community group (e.g., public weigh in, weight report card, fasting event to raise money for charity).	☐	☐	☐
Participating in sports and activities that focus on body weight, shape, and size (e.g., gymnastics, ballet, wrestling, modeling).	☐	☐	☐
Experiencing a change in friendship or peer group.	☑	☐	☐
Going to a new school, dropping out of school, school problems.	☑	☐	☐
Personal Concerns			
Dieting to lose weight or change body shape.	☐	☐	☐
Worrying about a social event with a focus on body weight, shape, and size (e.g., school fashion show, prom, swim party).	☐	☐	☐
Starting pubertal development before peer group.	☐	☐	☐
Breaking up with friends, girlfriends, boyfriends, or partner.	☐	☐	☐
Changing or losing a job.	☐	☐	☐
Not making a team.	☐	☐	☐
Family Concerns			
Family members constantly dieting.	☑	☐	☐
Experiencing financial stress in family.	☑	☐	☐
Increasing family conflict.	☑	☐	☐
Moving to a new town or neighborhood.	☐	☐	☐
Parents separating or divorcing.	☐	☐	☐
Close family member moving out or dying.	☐	☐	☐

CHAPTER 4

What Factors Cause the Increasing Prevalence of Eating Disorders?

There is no one reason or cause that explains why eating disorders have become so common in our society. Similarly, there is no one reason or cause that explains why one person gets an eating disorder while another does not. However, there are several factors that can be linked to the increase in eating disorders since the late 1960s.

Biological Factors

A female's body undergoes more natural physical changes throughout a lifetime than a male's body. For instance, there are increases in fat deposition at puberty, changes in shape and weight during pregnancy, and increases in weight during menopause. As a result, women tend to be more conscious of weight change and body image.

Hormonal Abnormalities

Aside from natural biological factors, some medical scientists have looked for biological abnormalities common to adolescents with eating disorders that will explain why some young people develop eating disorders and others do not.

Some candidates for such biological factors have included problems with hormones that affect appetite and the hypothalamus (seat of appetite in the brain); problems with chemicals in the brain that affect mood and the olfactory organs (parts of the head and brain related to smell); and problems with endogenous opioids (pleasure and satisfaction hormones in the brain). Further investigations, however, have not clearly delineated the role that each of these candidates plays in being a cause or result of an eating disorder.

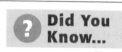
Did You Know...

• Of those children with anorexia nervosa who are 13 years old or younger, approximately 1 in 5 are boys, 4 in 5 are girls.

• About 1 in 10 teens and adults with anorexia are males, 9 in 10 are females.

• Bulimia nervosa is also more widespread among female than among male adolescents and adults. Why is this so? One possibility is biological factors. Another is sociocultural.

Genetic Vulnerabilities

Recently, research interest has turned to genetic factors that may contribute to the development of an eating disorder. No one gene appears to be responsible for anorexia nervosa or bulimia nervosa, though a number of genes may contribute to a person's vulnerability, given certain environmental conditions.

These genetic vulnerabilities to developing eating disorders are further supported by research studies showing that eating disorders cluster in families. This clustering cannot be entirely attributable to a particular family environment.

Many aspects of our culture are likely to be particularly difficult for people who have more than the average tendency toward perfectionism, obsessiveness, depression, or anxiety. For example, imagine a teenage girl who is going through all the changes of adolescence and who is also very socially sensitive. She is easily humiliated and very anxious about saying the right thing. She becomes overwhelmed with tension when in a group situation. Suppose she is also perfectionistic, always dissatisfied with things she says in a group setting and, therefore, often negatively interprets the facial expressions and behaviors of her peers.

To solve this problem, she tries to lose weight, having learned from our culture that changing body shape can be a solution to lack of confidence and will lead to being accepted

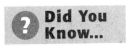

Did You Know...

- Several biological factors that were once thought to cause eating disorders are actually effects of them. For example, hormonal changes associated with loss of menses are caused by weight loss in anorexia nervosa.

- Malnutrition can have an impact on the hormones that affect growth, resulting in growth failure.

CASE STUDY Susan

After Susan's parents' experience on the eating disorder ward, they were curious about adolescent eating disorders and began to read about them. They wanted to understand why adolescents develop eating disorders.

However, reading about eating disorders made them very anxious because they saw a lot of their daughter in these books. She was a female adolescent who had been dieting. She was a high achiever and was always very focused and successful at whatever she did. She liked things to be perfect, and if they couldn't be, it was very upsetting to her.

What was really upsetting to her mother was that Susan's first cousin had been diagnosed with anorexia nervosa when she was 14 years old. Susan's mom remembered that this was a family secret...no one ever talked about it. Her cousin recovered from the eating disorder but this took many years. Susan's mother was very concerned after reading the material about eating disorders. Susan's father remained confident that Susan would be just fine...all she had to do was eat!

continued on page 51

by peers. If our teenage girl tries losing weight as a solution, she will likely be admired for her willpower, envied for her slimness, and as a result will feel in control. So the next time she feels anxious, humiliated, or out of control, she will focus with greater resolve to control her eating more perfectly. Doing this in the past helped her feel better.

Sociocultural Factors

Genetic vulnerabilities to perfectionism, obsessive compulsive behavior, anxiety, or depression may only be vulnerabilities for eating disorders in cultures, such as ours, that encourage perfectionistic standards and place an obsessive focus on appearance, connecting feeling better, being better, and being more confident with weight loss, appetite control, and having the 'right' kind of body.

Identity Transitions
Social and cultural identity transitions may play a part in the development of eating disorders among women. Certain sociocultural factors affect girls more than boys. Appearance is more central to how females are valued and therefore more central to a girl's self-esteem.

Another factor, especially in North America, is that the economic role of women and, therefore, their sense of identity has changed more frequently than the roles of males. During World War II, for example, women were pulled from their roles at home to replace men in factory jobs, but then went home again when the soldiers returned after the war and immigrants arrived in large numbers.

Women's role in our culture has also changed with the advent of the feminist movement in the 1960s. Girls growing up since then have enjoyed new opportunities but, in many cases, have been expected to maintain their traditional role in the home. The double pressure of maintaining a job and a home may have an impact on eating behavior.

Ideal Body Image
Our culture directs messages to females that make them more likely to be dissatisfied with their bodies and urges girls and women to engage in dieting behaviors.

Eating disorders have not always been common. Since

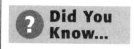
Did You Know...

• Researchers speculate that vulnerability to eating disorders may be connected to such genetic traits as a tendency to be a perfectionist and a tendency to be obsessive compulsive, or they may be connected to the brain chemicals that affect depression and anxiety levels.

• These genetic traits are all known risk factors for eating disorders.

FIJI STUDY

Cultures, such as contemporary Western culture, that have a very thin body ideal (or promote food restriction for some other reason) and are in the process of changing in a way that affects female roles appear prone to developing eating disorders among women.

A study conducted in Fiji between 1995 and 1998 shows how the combination of thin body ideals and role transition for females can be very problematic. In Fiji, a rounded female body shape had always been valued. Traditionally, the economy had been based on farming and fishing, but during the 1990s, it underwent a transition to an industry-based economy. Dieting was rare in Fiji. There was no television until 1995, when two channels began broadcasting Western dramas, comedies, and advertising.

By 1998, the culture had changed dramatically: 69% of the young women in the study reported dieting to lose weight and 74% reported feeling too big or too fat. Three times as many girls as previously were in the high-risk group for eating disorders. While there had been no reports of self-induced vomiting in 1995, 12% of the girls reported this behavior in 1998. In their interviews, the young women said they did not want to be "fat" like their mothers; they felt fatter when watching television shows; and they wanted to have the lifestyle and the body shapes they saw on the television.

There seems to be a relationship between being exposed to Western society and developing eating disorders, among females in particular. This may occur when families or individuals emigrate from a non-Western to a Western society or where the society is making a transition from a traditional to a Westernized culture, as in Fiji. What happens to young women in these transitional societies only magnifies what is happening in Western culture itself.

the 1960s, there has been a sharp increase in the incidence of bulimia nervosa. During this period of time, the media has been portraying a very thin body type as an ideal shape for girls and women. In fact, this so-called ideal body is associated with a significantly lower body fat level that is unhealthy for growing and developing children and adolescents. This ideal body has increased the pressure on girls and women to diet. Since dieting contributes to the development of bulimia nervosa, we can say that the high rate of bulimia nervosa has come about in relation to unrealistic body ideals in Western culture.

During the same time, there has also been a significant increase in anorexia nervosa. Whether this increase in anorexia nervosa is associated with improvement in the ability of our health-care professionals to identify anorexia nervosa or whether there is a true increase in the disorder among adolescents is not clear, but historical trends in ideal body images suggest the disorder is growing.

Puberty Paradox

Before the onset of puberty, boys and girls have approximately the same amount of body fat. At puberty, boys' bodies develop greater muscle and less fat, while girls' bodies tend to increase in fat. This increase in fat is necessary for normal menstrual periods. Our culture has put girls at odds with their own developmental process by idealizing the thin body type for females. Young girls are set up to dislike the changes that come with puberty. Normal increases in the amount of body fat may be perceived as getting fat, which may lead adolescent girls to look for ways to make themselves thinner.

Despite these normal physical changes, there is continued pressure to be thin and toned at every age. Dieting is probably the most common practice adopted by girls for this purpose. In fact, many adolescents with eating disorders begin by going on a diet.

Insecurity

This 'culture of thinness' obviously contributes to the increased prevalence of eating disorders. Other less obvious aspects of our culture also play an important role.

Insecurity, for example, can be a factor in eating disorders. Insecurity is created when the expectations that come with meeting certain standards are impossible to achieve, such as the standards of beauty portrayed on television, in movies, or in magazines. The advertising media associates images of beauty with being youthful. As the body ages, women cannot meet the expectation of remaining youthful in appearance. Thin women are also frequently portrayed as being happy, content, and in control, regardless of how stressful their lives may be.

Food advertisements are another source of insecurity. On the one hand, they encourage women to indulge themselves, and on the other, they caution women to take control of themselves by eating less. There does not seem to be one consistent message that supports the need for girls and women to nourish themselves consistently.

These messages tend to leave teens feeling that their bodies are not as they should be and that they are not living their lives properly according to the impossible standards presented to them. Such insecurity can lead girls to experience a decrease in their self-esteem during adolescence, which may put them at higher risk for developing an eating disorder.

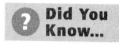

Did You Know...

● Anorexia nervosa was first identified in the late 1800s when people believed that eating very little was "ladylike" and that it contributed to spiritual purity.

● Since the 1960s, the ideal body shape for women has become increasingly thinner.

● Until the 1960s, research reveals that female models and actors weighed 7% less than the average woman, but by the 1970s, female models and actors weighed 15% less than the average woman.

CASE STUDY Martha

After Martha and her parents went to a psychoeducation group to learn more about eating disorders, they started to feel really vulnerable. Everywhere they looked, they noticed messages supporting or even encouraging young people and adults to be thin. The television was full of these messages. Most actors were thin! If there was an actor that was fat, they were always the brunt of horrible "fat jokes."

At work, a colleague of Martha's mother told her she looked great because she had "lost some weight." This comment brought Martha's mother to tears. She had not intentionally lost weight. Her weight loss was a result of worrying about her daughter. Martha's mother recognized that before this eating disorder had entered their family's life, such a comment would have made her feel good. After all, in our weight-obsessed world, any weight loss, no matter how much or how it is accomplished, is a good thing. However, under the current circumstances, losing weight was not a good thing.

continued on page 103

Perfectionism

Insecurity can also lead to perfectionism as young people strive to meet these standards and match the ideal body image. We know that perfectionism is often part of an eating disorder. In many ways, our society and culture encourage perfectionism.

Perfecting an image has been made possible by contemporary technology. Magazine photographs of women are retouched and imperfections are airbrushed away. Television also eliminates imperfections, as Marshall McLuhan pointed out, because television images have low definition. As a result, even when the original object being televised is flawed, the televised image looks smooth and clean. When we compare actual objects and people with televised images of them, we start thinking there are imperfections in the originals.

Such images become the standard for what real things and people should look like, even if young women would like to think that inner beauty is more important than outer beauty and that beauty can be found in round bodies, wrinkled faces, and other ordinary human qualities. They are told by the media and by their peers that what they do is "never good enough." They begin to see themselves as 'less than.'

Control

Our culture places a high value on being 'in control,' leaving many young women who are not in control feeling like they do not measure up or fit in. Being hesitant, confused, or unsure are seen as signs of weakness.

For adolescents, this situation is particularly difficult. At this stage in their lives, they are naturally unsure of themselves, in the process of developing a sense of identity and undergoing major body-related changes. They need to be able to experiment and make mistakes, but they need the approval of their peers more than they ever will again. They are learning to take responsibility for their lives and learning to negotiate relationships with other people. There is probably no other time of life when people are feeling less perfect than during their adolescence. Yet teens in our culture are pressured to appear to be both confident and in control.

Parents may add to this pressure by wanting their children to reflect the characteristics of a personality type our culture celebrates more than others — that is, the outgoing, confident, group-oriented leader. More reserved children who are content to involve themselves in quieter activities are not valued as highly by our culture. Parents of such children may find themselves pressured to direct their children into activities that emphasize characteristics their children don't have. Such children may feel the need to perform to fulfill a picture of themselves that isn't real.

Increasingly, our schools also put pressure on students to do better academically in order to get into the 'right' high school so they can get into the 'right' university and ultimately get the 'right' job. In some elementary schools, students

> **? Did You Know...**
>
> • By not allowing teens to develop *real* confidence, our culture puts them at risk of looking for ways to *appear* confident and in control. For girls, and to a lesser extent, boys, reducing body fat is seen as a way to accomplish this.

CASE STUDY Brad

Brad's father was concerned about how easily little comments would affect his supersensitive son. Everyone regarded Brad as a sweet, hard-working boy with a good heart. Everywhere Brad looked, people were talking about the importance of being healthy and living a healthy lifestyle. In turn,

Brad took these messages to the absolute extreme.

If being fat meant that he was unhealthy, then he was going to achieve a healthy weight…a healthy weight meant achieving the lowest possible weight on the scale.

continued on page 128

can now get more than 100% on a test by earning bonus points. Thus, children are not always given guidance on how to recognize realistic limits to help them identify what they should reasonably expect of themselves.

False Logic

Girls are more often socialized by their families to be more attentive to the feelings and needs of others than are boys. This occurs in a culture that also places a high value on independence. Girls are more likely to avoid bringing forward their own needs when stressful circumstances create pressure on them. For instance, a girl whose family is preoccupied with a parent's or sibling's illness may see that there is little attention available for her and will deny her own needs to demonstrate her strength and independence in order to help out her family. Dieting and losing weight can then 'help' the girl because it makes her feel not only like she's increased her attractiveness and value, but also that she's strong and independent. She's conquered her appetite and shown that she can 'do without.'

Family

Over the last 30 years, there has been much speculation about how families might contribute to eating disorders. At one time, it was suggested that certain types of families were more at risk for having a child with an eating disorder. For example, families with a child suffering from anorexia nervosa seemed to be more tightly controlled and highly organized. Families with a child with bulimia nervosa seemed to be more chaotic, conflicted, and critical.

Still, some risk factors have been associated with families, notably in families that have an excessive concern about weight and appearance with a great focus on dieting; in families where children show extreme discomfort in discussing problems with parents; and in immigrant families having difficulty adapting to Western values.

The eating disorder can have a serious impact on the health of the family. Families commonly experience conflict, relationship difficulties, and even marital difficulties.

Given the significant effect of our sociocultural environment on adolescents, it is important for families to provide a caring, safe, and supportive environment that offers an alternative to a culture that over-values a thin body image and 'having it all together.'

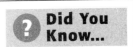

Did You Know...

• Few health-care professionals believe that a specific family type will cause an eating disorder.

• Research indicates that adolescents with eating disorders come from all different types of family.

CHAPTER 5

What Is Normal Adolescent Development?

When you are worrying about a child who shows signs of having an eating disorder, you can sometimes lose focus on what constitutes normal adolescent growth and development. So many things seem to be going awry with your child that you can't imagine what is right. Understanding how children and adolescents are supposed to develop in body and mind offers a model to use in diagnosing an eating disorder and monitoring the effect of treatments. Once diagnosis of an eating order is confirmed, your aim is to help your child restore normal eating behavior and, ultimately, normal growth and development — physically, psychologically, and emotionally.

During adolescence, significant changes occur in both the body and mind of a young person, referred to as biological and psychosocial changes. While it is impossible to separate the biological changes from the psychosocial ones completely, we will do so for the ease of explanation.

What Is Adolescence?

Adolescence is a time of major physical, psychological, and emotional development. The word "adolescence" comes from the Latin word *adolescere*, which means to "grow up," and the Latin root *esco*, which means "becoming." This period is when children "become" or develop into adults. Changes that the adolescent experiences during this time of life are second only to the dramatic growth and development that occur during a baby's first year of life.

We commonly consider the first physical changes of puberty as the beginning of adolescence, but defining the completion of adolescence and transition into adulthood is more difficult. Is it the time when physical growth is completed? Is it the time when young people leave the parental home? Is it the time when financial independence is achieved or education completed?

During our era, going through adolescence has become a lengthy process. Years ago, girls had their first period at an average age of 16 and shortly thereafter had their own families. Boys went out to work once they had the physical strength to take on the family-provider role. Society expected children to become adults over a very short period of time. Now, society expects these changes to occur over a much longer time frame. This enables a smoother transition from childhood to adulthood, and enables us, the parents and caregivers, to adjust to the changes our children go through.

Puberty now starts earlier, at times at the end of the first decade of life, and adolescence may end only during the third decade of life, after education has been completed, financial independence achieved, and a mature personality formed.

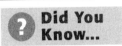

Did You Know...

- The age of the first menstrual period dropped from 16 to 12.5 years of age in the past century. This is mainly due to improved nutrition, but other factors might also contribute to this change.

Puberty (Sexual Maturity)

Puberty is the physical process that brings a child to full adulthood. The trigger for the onset of the hormonal changes that begin the pubertal process is unclear, however. Many factors play a role in determining the age of onset of puberty, including the age at which the young person's parents and siblings began puberty, as well as their own ethnicity, nutritional status, and emotional and physical well-being.

There is also a wide range of normal in terms of age of onset of puberty in both females and males, as well as between individuals of the same gender.

In order to accurately describe the stage of physical development or puberty of the young person, doctors and nurses revert to a scale known as the Sexual Maturity Rating (SMR) scale. This rating scale allows doctors and nurses to track the physical changes of puberty in each young person, and identify when the various events of puberty are proceeding in a predictable, normal fashion and when they are not.

SEXUAL MATURITY RATING (SMR)

The SMR is a scale that categorizes changes in breast and pubic hair development in females, and pubic hair, testicle, and penis development in males. It assigns a number from 1 through 5 to these physical changes, with 1 representing no evidence of puberty and 5 representing full adult maturity.

If you are concerned about your child's physical development through puberty, consult your family doctor or pediatrician.

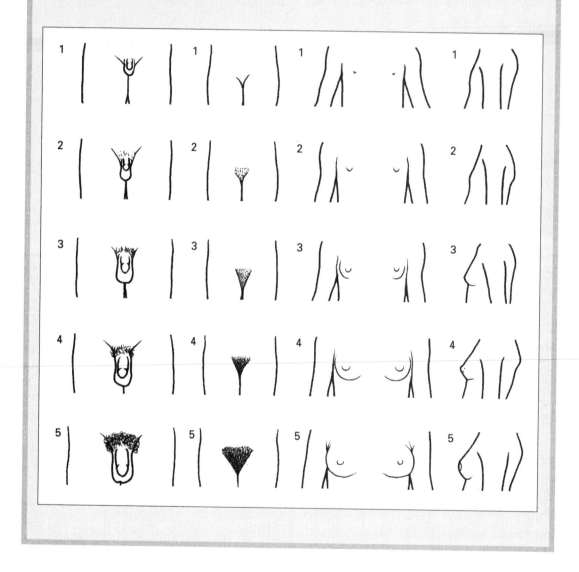

CASE STUDY Jessica

I often wonder…why me? Why did I get this eating disorder? I think things started getting bad when I was 9 years old. I was the first of all of my friends to get breasts and curves, and everyone teased me about it. Then on top of everything…I got my period. It was terrible. I am sure I was the first to get my period. Of course no one talked about it.

I was so upset about getting my period that my mom took me to my doctor to see if I was normal. The doctor said, "That's what happens when you are chubby." I was humiliated. All the other girls were slim and straight, why did I have to have curves? Why did I have to develop breasts? And, why did I have to get my period? The others kids constantly teased me about by body weight and shape. They were really cruel and no one wanted to be my friend. I felt all alone and like I was the worst person on the planet.

So, I decided to lose weight so I could get rid of all this fat. Hey, maybe I would even lose my periods! I went on a major diet.

continued on page 69

Puberty in Females

Before the first physical signs of puberty can be seen, the hormonal system (the system that regulates physical growth and sexual maturation) has already been activated. This produces changes in the internal organs of the female reproductive system, including growth and changes to the uterus and ovaries. These organs, located in the pelvis, cannot be seen and therefore cannot be used as indicators that puberty has started. Instead, breast development, changes in body and pubic hair (secondary sexual characteristics), and the onset of the menstrual period all serve as signs that help to assess the progression of puberty in females.

Age of Onset

Doctors and nurses track these physical changes using the SMR scale. It is normal for the physical signs of puberty to start any time between 7.5 and 12 years of age. Having these signs before 7.5 years, or having no signs of puberty at all by 13 years of age, should be discussed with a doctor who is knowledgeable about growth and development. The whole pubertal process can take up to 4 years to complete.

There is an expected pattern for the changes of puberty seen in females. Initially, the breasts start to grow, called breast budding. This is followed by the appearance of scarce hair in the pubic region that gradually takes the form of

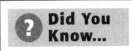

Did You Know…

● Females usually grow 8 to 12 inches or 20 to 30 centimeters during puberty. Most of their growth is completed by the age of 14.

● A marked weight gain is also expected during this time. Doubling of weight within a few years of the onset of puberty is a normal, expected occurrence.

coarse, adult-type pubic hair. The time when adolescent girls grow the most, referred to as their growth spurt, usually occurs relatively early in puberty, shortly after breast budding and the first appearance of scant pubic hair.

Menstruation

Only after the growth spurt has taken place will most females have their first menstrual period. This occurs about 2.5 years from the start of breast budding. Growth then slows down, but still continues for another year or two. Usually girls grow no more than 2 inches or 5 centimeters after their first period. The menstrual cycle may initially be irregular, sometimes with no period at all for a few months, or sometimes with bleeding every 2 to 3 weeks. Bleeding may be heavy or light, with or without cramps. If an irregular menstrual pattern continues beyond the first year or the bleeding is very heavy, you should consult a doctor.

> **Q:** My daughter is 15 years old and her height is 5'0" (152 cm). I am 5'5" (165 cm) and my husband is 5'8" (173 cm). She has been menstruating for three years. I was told that she probably won't grow anymore? Is that true?
>
> **A:** Yes, girls almost reach their full adult height when they get their first menstrual period. Usually girls grow no more than 2 inches or 5 centimeters after their first period.

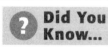

Did You Know...

• Boys can grow 4 to 5 inches or 10 to 12 centimeters in one year during their growth spurt.

• Girls usually grow only 3 to 4 inches or 8 to 10 centimeters in one year during that time of rapid growth.

Shape Changes

Weight gain and increase in height are also accompanied by a change in the shape of the female body, with widening of the hip and thigh areas. Total body fat increases from about 8% in childhood to a range of 20% to 22% in the average adult female. This change in body composition is due mainly to the increased levels of the female sex hormone estrogen.

Parents and girls entering puberty need to be aware of these expected yet relatively rapid changes in body size and shape. This awareness might ease possible anxiety around the normal weight gain that occurs as a natural progression of puberty.

CASE STUDY Susan

Susan noticed that her breasts were getting larger and slightly tender now that she had put on some weight. They had shrunk when she had lost the weight. She was upset at the sight of her breasts getting larger…that meant that she might even get her period soon!

That also meant that she was getting fat. Her distress at getting fat was overwhelming — she would have to do something to lose weight. She had to get out of the hospital.

continued on page 67

Q: **My 13-year-old daughter still hasn't had her first period. All her friends have their period. Should I be worried that there may something wrong with her? I got my menstrual period when I was 13.**

A: There is no one age at which all girls will get their menstrual period. There are some important facts that will help you predict when your daughter may get her period. First, a girl usually gets her menstrual period about 2.5 years after her breasts start to develop. In addition, girls traditionally start to menstruate within one year of when their mothers started to menstruate.

Puberty in Males

There are several differences in the physical changes of puberty between males and females.

Age of Onset

Males start puberty about a year and a half later than females, usually between 9.5 and 13.5 years of age. Unlike females, the changes in their sexual organs, the penis and testicles, can be observed. These changes, along with the development of body and facial hair, the protuberance of the Adam's apple, and the deepening of the male's voice (secondary sex characteristics) may serve as markers for the onset and progression of puberty in males. The SMR scale is used for males, as it is for females, to better track the stages of development each young male goes through.

Q: My son is 13 years old. He looks quite young compared to his other male friends. Some of his friends are looking more like men. Should I be concerned?

A: There is great variation in the age at which puberty starts and the speed with which it progresses for male and female adolescents. Healthy adolescents of the same age may look very different from one another, as shown in these representations of healthy 13-year-old adolescents.

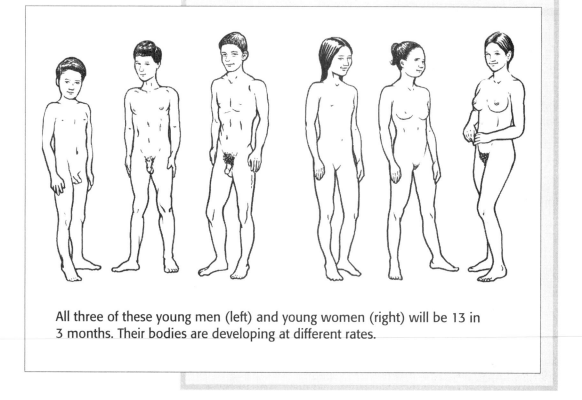

All three of these young men (left) and young women (right) will be 13 in 3 months. Their bodies are developing at different rates.

Sexual Development

Like females, males also follow a predictable pattern of pubertal development. Puberty generally starts with the darkening and roughening of the scrotum (the skin covering the testes), followed by an increase in the volume of the testes, and the appearance of fine hair in the pubic area that gradually changes to coarse, adult-type pubic hair. As well, the penis first grows in length and then in width. At this stage the boy experiences his first ejaculation of sperm, sometimes referred to as a wet dream or spermarche.

Normal Growth in Height and Weight

Only relatively late in puberty does the male have a rapid increase in height or growth spurt. This is usually after an SMR of 4 is achieved, when the changes in pubic hair growth and distribution and development of the penis and testicles are almost complete.

Growth not only occurs in the trunk area, but also in the extremities. The first place to elongate is the foot, followed by the calves and the thighs. A similar pattern happens in the upper limbs, with the hands elongating first and then the arms. The growth of the trunk, with widening of the chest and shoulders, happens last. This leads to a transient disproportion of the limbs and the trunk, which contributes to the characteristic clumsiness often seen during adolescence.

Shape Changes

Similar to what is observed in girls, the boy's body changes not only in height and weight but also in shape. The male muscle mass increases significantly during puberty, mostly due to the effect of male hormones known as androgens. Facial and body hair also appear during puberty under the stimulation of these hormones. The timing and progression of hair growth vary significantly between individuals. Usually hair under the arms (axillary hair) appears when facial hair is observed, and chest hair appears late in puberty. The amount of hair on the face and body of males is dependent not only on hormonal levels, but also on the ethnic and family background of the individual.

Growth Curves

Health-care professionals use growth charts to monitor height (stature) and weight changes in children and adolescents. Normal growth patterns are established by sampling a large number of your people. Abnormal growth may indicate a medical problem, such as an eating disorder. A return to a normal growth pattern in young people with an eating disorder may show the effects of treatment and the progress of recovery. Ask your family doctor or pediatrician to plot your child's growth curve and maintain growth charts for your child. They are valuable for diagnosing and treating an eating disorder.

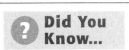
Did You Know...

• Most boys continue to grow at least until they are 16 years of age, with some continuing their growth until 19 years of age and older.

• At the end of puberty males are generally taller than females. This is due mainly to the greater and longer growth spurt males experience in comparison to females.

Male Children and Adolescents

Stature-for-Age and Weight-for-Age percentiles for boys, from 2 to 20 years, so that you can track your child's growth curve.

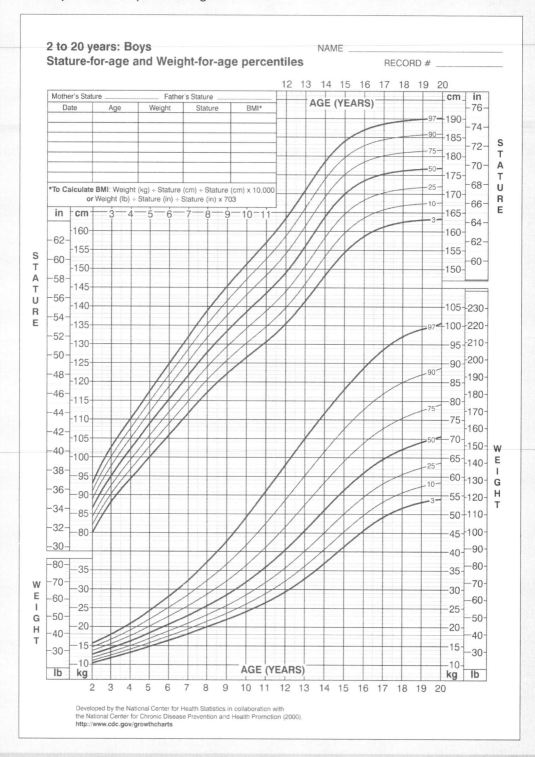

2 to 20 years: Boys
Stature-for-age and Weight-for-age percentiles

NAME

RECORD #

Developed by the National Center for Health Statistics in collaboration with the National Center for Chronic Disease Prevention and Health Promotion (2000).
http://www.cdc.gov/growthcharts

Female Children and Adolescents

Stature-for-Age and Weight-for-Age percentiles for girls, from 2 to 20 years, so that you can track your child's growth curve.

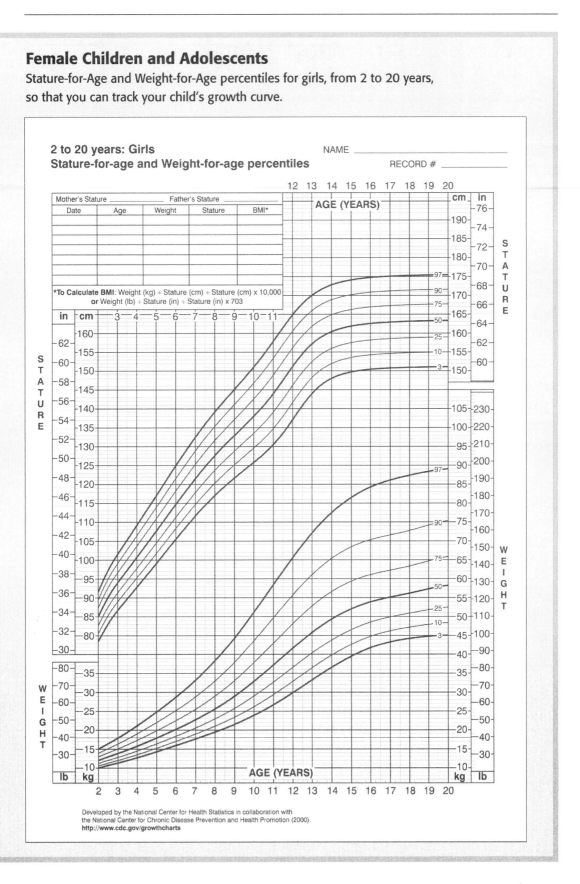

2 to 20 years: Girls
Stature-for-age and Weight-for-age percentiles

NAME _____

RECORD # _____

Mother's Stature _____ Father's Stature _____

Date	Age	Weight	Stature	BMI*

*To Calculate BMI: Weight (kg) ÷ Stature (cm) ÷ Stature (cm) x 10,000
or Weight (lb) ÷ Stature (in) ÷ Stature (in) x 703

AGE (YEARS)

Developed by the National Center for Health Statistics in collaboration with
the National Center for Chronic Disease Prevention and Health Promotion (2000).
http://www.cdc.gov/growthcharts

Nutrition Needs

For female and male adolescents to achieve their full growth potential in height and weight during this time, proper nutrition is required. Minerals and vitamins also play an important role in this healthy growth. The intake of all the required elements in food can be accomplished only through a well-balanced diet that includes a variety of foods.

Growth occurs in the internal organs of males and females during puberty, as well as in their blood system. For the blood system, iron is an important nutrient. Once females start having menstrual periods, they lose small amounts of blood monthly, and if not enough iron is supplemented through their diet, this loss may cause iron deficiency anemia. This could have an impact on the physical and mental well-being of the adolescent.

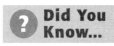 **Did You Know...**

• The amount of blood actually doubles during puberty, requiring a sufficient amount of iron to assist in creating many new blood cells to help carry oxygen to the growing body.

• During puberty, the bones need more calcium than ever in order to become strong for life. This unique growth of bones is regulated by hormones and requires vitamin D, estrogen, and calcium.

Psychosocial Growth and Development

Proper growth and development during puberty are also influenced by the psychological and emotional well-being of the adolescent. Children who are deprived emotionally or are under a great deal of stress may not achieve their full growth potential.

The psychosocial development of adolescents is often described as the process leading them to master changes in certain areas of their lives. Parents, teachers, and other careproviders need to understand the expected psychosocial development of adolescents to reduce the stress and, at times, frustration adults feel while caring for young people going through their development. This knowledge may also help parents and other adults relate to young people in a more caring and accepting way, allowing more autonomy, yet ensuring the safety of the young person.

Onset of Adolescent Psychosocial Development

There is great variation between individuals in the time of onset of psychosocial development, as well as the speed with which these changes occur. Each adolescent has different life circumstances and responds differently to challenges and opportunities. The process of psychosocial growth is not always continuous — the changes may sometimes occur over a short period of time and, in other instances, may take a longer time to progress. At yet other times it may even look as if the adolescent is going backwards in psychosocial maturity, temporarily regressing to more childish behavior that might seem surprising for the person's age. This shifting between types of behavior and stages of maturity is quite normal for the period of adolescence and depends on the many factors playing a role in the young person's life at that particular stage.

> **? Did You Know...**
>
> • Not all individuals reach full maturity in every aspect of their psychosocial development at the same time — some may even remain relatively immature in certain areas throughout their lifetime. This, too, is not necessarily abnormal.

DEVELOPMENTAL TASKS

The various psychosocial changes that the young person undergoes are often referred to by health-care professionals as developmental tasks.

- Becoming independent from parents.

- Adopting the values, social rules, and lifestyle of the young person's peer group (for example, wearing similar cloths and speaking in the same manner as friends).

- Paying more attention to the physical changes that occur during puberty, usually ending with acceptance of the new, adult body.

- Establishing a personal identity with respect to moral and ethical issues, as well as having career goals (the "who am I" and "what do I want to do when I grow up" phase).

THREE STAGES OF ADOLESCENCE

Generally speaking, the period of adolescence can be divided into three stages with respect to psychological and emotional development: early, mid, and late adolescence. Each individual goes through these three phases, but not necessarily at the exact ages suggested here. No one individual experiences these stages in precisely the same way as another does.

Early Adolescence (10 to 13 years)

Independence: The physical changes that occur in this early stage of adolescence often go hand in hand with the adolescent's wish for independence. Compared to when they were younger, there is usually less interest in their parents' activities, greater realization that the parent is not always perfect, and a search for other significant figures to look up to besides parents.

Mood Swings: It is not uncommon for the young adolescent to experience mood swings.

Questioning Authority: The young person may start to be 'difficult' at home and school performance may decline. This may be because the early adolescent has begun to question authority and look more to peer groups for support and validation than to parents and teachers.

Friendships: Most close friends at this early stage of adolescence are from the same sex, but there may be some contact with the opposite sex.

Body Image: As the young person's body goes through the physical changes of puberty, there is increasing preoccupation with body image. Young adolescents spend more time critically looking at their bodies, questioning their looks, and comparing themselves to friends.

Sexual Awakening: Sexual feelings may have begun even before the onset of puberty, but there is an expected increased interest in sex during early adolescence. This usually starts with the exploration of the young person's own body, including masturbation.

Thinking Ability: The adolescent's cognitive abilities start to mature significantly during this early stage of development. The concrete, child-like way of thinking about things that can only be seen, heard, or sensed develops into a more sophisticated ability to reason and think abstractly. As well, verbal communication skills improve. There may be an increase in daydreaming, setting of unrealistic life goals, and overall idealism about the world.

Mid Adolescence (14 to 16 years)

Increasing Independence: Mid adolescence is often characterized by the adolescent's struggle for increasing independence. Conflicts with parents often become more common, and the peer group plays an even greater role in the young person's life. The increasing need for independence may lead to greater separation from parents, but may also strengthen the young person's social skills and lead to a drive for excellence in academics, music, or sports.

Peer Pressure: Adolescents going through this developmental stage often take on the peer group's codes, style, and values. In fact, it is not uncommon to see groups of adolescents who dress and act alike in as many ways as possible during mid adolescence. Although peer pressure is almost always a major force during this stage of development, each adolescent responds differently to it. Some respond in a very positive way and do well, while others may experience difficulties.

Appearance: As many of the pubertal changes have already occurred by mid adolescence, particularly in females, young people may become preoccupied with trying to make their bodies more attractive. It is common, though not always healthy, for adolescents to diet or be involved in bodybuilding in an attempt to improve how they feel about themselves and to try to appear more attractive to others. Now is the time for all caregivers to advise adolescents about a healthy, balanced way of eating and exercising in order to prevent unwanted consequences from both undereating and overexercising.

Dating: Adolescents often start dating during this period, with some exploring sexual relationships with their partners.

Intellectual Growth: The intellectual ability to reason and think abstractly continues to develop during mid adolescence. This is often illustrated by the young person's increasing capacity to perceive future implications of current acts and decisions. Like younger adolescents, feelings of having ultimate power and being immortal are still common at this stage of development. A thought like 'I can do anything and nothing wrong can happen to me' is not uncommon at this stage of development. For some, this may lead to risk-taking behaviors, such as substance use and abuse, unprotected sexual intercourse, or careless driving.

Late Adolescence (17 years and older)

Accepting Limitations: This phase of development often brings to a close the previous struggles for identity and separation from parents that are seen in the earlier adolescent years. With a supportive environment, the restlessness that is typical for earlier stages of adolescence is gradually calmed by the young person's ability to compromise and acknowledge limits of self, parents, and society in general.

Growing Confidence: The young person becomes more confident and is, therefore, more willing to seek parental advice and even adopt many of their values – often the same ones that they had rejected earlier in their development. It is not uncommon, though, for some adolescents to follow a completely different path in life than their parents in order to make the separation from their families more distinct.

Body Image: The physical changes of puberty are usually completed by this stage of development and young people become more accepting of their own body.

Relationships: The peer group and its values become less important, and there is more interest and investment in developing closer, intimate relationships.

Cognitive Development: Intellectual functioning continues to mature to adult levels, with educational and occupational goals becoming more realistic.

CHAPTER 6

How Do You Identify a Child or Adolescent with an Eating Disorder?

There are common signs and symptoms of eating disorders in physical appearance and daily behavior that enable diagnosis. Recognizing these signs and symptoms at an early stage in the development of the disorder will certainly aid in treatment and recovery. But recognizing these indications is not always easy.

An eating disorder usually develops slowly over time, making it difficult for parents to detect changes in their child's appearance. Adolescents tend to spend less time with their families and more time with their friends, leaving less opportunity for parents to interact and talk with them. Teens are not always willing to bring personal issues to their parents or discuss any difficulties they might be having. This can make parents feel guilty for not having noticed that something was wrong sooner.

As parents, you need to watch your children, listen to them, and talk to them to see and hear if they are developing an eating disorder. While the signs and symptoms of eating disorders presented here may not confirm that your child has an eating disorder — some of the signs and symptoms associated with eating disorders can also be seen in other medical or psychiatric conditions — they, nevertheless, provide a starting point.

As parents, you are the expert when it comes to the health and well-being of your children. If you see any indication that your child might have an eating disorder, then you should make an appointment with your family doctor or pediatrician. If the eating disorder is not treated, it can become life threatening.

 Did You Know...

● In a recent survey of girls aged 12 to18 years, over 25% of them had significant symptoms of an eating disorder.

● Another survey showed that 30% of girls 10 to 14 years old were trying to lose weight.

● By the age of 18 years, 80% of girls of normal height and weight reported that they would like to weigh less.

Physical Appearance

Among changes in the physical appearance of a child or adolescent developing an eating disorder are weight reduction or fluctuation, lack of growth, and delay in puberty.

Weight Loss, Gain, or Fluctuations

Childhood and adolescence is a time of intense growth. Healthy children and adolescents should not be losing weight. In fact, they should be gaining weight as they grow in height and progress through puberty. Internal organs, bones, muscle, and fat proportions change during puberty. This is part of normal development. Adolescents should continue to grow and gain weight throughout this time until they have finished puberty and reached their adult size and shape. Any significant or unexpected weight loss or repeated, large weight fluctuations should be checked by your doctor.

Anorexia Nervosa

Children and adolescents with anorexia nervosa can often lose a large amount of weight in a short period of time. Take this sign seriously. If your child severely restricts food intake, this may lead to rapid weight loss and medical problems. Weight loss may initially go unnoticed because young people with anorexia nervosa often wear baggy or layered clothing in an attempt to hide their weight loss, to conceal what they perceive as 'fat', and to help them stay warm. Young people with eating disorders often feel cold compared to healthy teenagers who are at normal weight. This weight loss may become more obvious over the summer months when teenagers start to wear lighter clothing. If you start to notice your child's backbone, ribs, collarbones, or cheekbones are sticking out, this indicates that there has been a significant loss in body fat.

Bulimia Nervosa

Children and adolescents with bulimia nervosa may have dramatic weight fluctuations due to their erratic eating behaviors. The adolescent's weight can rise and fall from one week to the next. Teenagers who binge or binge and purge can have these types of weight changes.

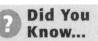 **Did You Know...**

- At peak growth, adolescent girls have an increase in weight of 18 pounds or 8 kilograms per year.

- At peak growth, adolescent males have an increase in weight of 20 pounds or 9 kilograms per year.

- Girls increase their body fat during puberty from 16% of body weight before puberty to 27% by the end of puberty. This is normal.

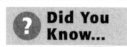

Did You Know...

• Growth during puberty accounts for 20% to 25% of adult height.

• Males have an average increase in height of 11 inches or 28 centimeters during puberty.

• Females have an average increase in height of 9.8 inches or 25 centimeters during puberty.

Lack of Growth

If you notice that your child has stopped growing in height at a time when other teenagers are starting or are in the midst of their growth spurt, discuss this with your child's doctor. Growth delay can be due to many factors, one of these being an eating disorder.

When an adolescent is malnourished and not eating enough, the body uses all the energy it gets just to keep working. The body is not able to build up muscles, bone, and energy stores, which results in a lack of growth. If this occurs for a long period of time, adolescents may end up being shorter than what they would have been if they did not have an eating disorder.

Your doctor should be measuring and recording your child's growth in weight and height. These measurements should be plotted on a growth curve, which shows the average rate and amount of growth in children and adolescents of different age groups and genders. Growth curves allow your doctor to record and follow the pattern of your child's growth in weight and height. This is the best way to detect a delay in height or a change in weight. If you are not sure that this is happening, ask your child's doctor.

Puberty and Menstruation

A number of factors determine the onset and ongoing process of puberty (including menstruation for girls). The development of an eating disorder can delay both the start and progression of puberty in both girls and boys.

Girls who have started their menstrual periods often lose them when they develop anorexia nervosa or have irregular menstrual periods if they develop bulimia nervosa. If your daughter loses her periods or if her periods become irregular after being regular for many months, you should be concerned and have this investigated by your doctor. If your daughter is on the oral contraceptive pill (OCP), she may still have menstrual periods as a result of the hormones in the OCP. The OCP can hide one of the tell-tale signs of anorexia nervosa — the loss of her menstrual periods.

Q: My 15-year-old daughter first got her periods when she was 13. She had her period every month. She would mark it down on her calendar. She would also ask me to purchase tampons and menstrual pads on a regular basis. Over the past few months, she hasn't asked me to buy her tampons or pads. When I asked her about this, she got upset. I have also noticed that she hasn't been eating much for breakfast. Could she have an eating disorder?

A: Irregular periods are common in girls who are just starting to menstruate; in fact, it may take up to 2 years for your daughter's menstrual period to become regular. In the meantime, she may skip a period or two or have an irregular menstrual cycle. Chronic illness, dramatic weight loss or gain, excessive or strenuous exercise, stress, hormone imbalance (for example, too much or not enough thyroid hormone), some types of contraception, certain medications, pregnancy, and eating disorders can cause menstrual irregularities or amenorrhea (absence of menstrual periods).

If you are concerned about your daughter's menstrual period, be sure to speak to your child about your concerns. You should encourage her to make an appointment with her doctor to assess the situation. Her doctor can help determine the cause of irregular or absent menstrual periods. The doctor will also explore other signs, symptoms, and behaviors if there is concern that your daughter is developing an eating disorder.

Other Physical Signs of Eating Disorders

Besides apparent abnormalities in weight, height, and puberty, there are other physical signs and symptoms of eating disorders. Consult your child's doctor if you detect any one these indications.

Yellow- or orange-tinged skin

This can be the result of eating an excessive amount of foods that contain carotene (such as carrots) but can also be the result of starvation. It is often most noticeable on the palm of the hands.

Thinning hair or hair that breaks easily

Hair growth is affected by malnutrition and becomes more brittle.

Growth of downy hair on back, stomach, or the side of the face

Called lanugo hair, this is a result of the body reacting to loss of body fat in an attempt to maintain body temperature.

Conjunctival hemorrhages

These are broken blood vessels in the whites of the eyes and can be a result of forceful vomiting in people who purge after eating.

Swollen glands and 'chipmunk cheeks' appearance

The parotid glands, found just below the ears, become enlarged in people who binge and purge.

Calluses or scars on the back of the hand

If adolescents stick their fingers down their throat in an attempt to cause vomiting, they may develop calluses (areas of hard skin) on the back of their hand, a condition known as Russell's sign.

Eating Behaviors

Adolescents and children developing eating disorders often undergo significant changes in their eating behavior, such as dieting for the first time, skipping meals, counting and measuring the fat and the caloric content of food, eating alone, purging, and exhibiting other unusual eating behaviors.

Dieting

Children and adolescents require a variety of healthy foods to keep their bodies growing and developing properly. Young people with eating disorders can diet to the point of starvation.

A young person with an eating disorder may start out with what appears to be an innocent diet for looking fit and healthy. Family and friends may even give positive reinforcement as the young person goes on a diet to become more healthy by losing weight. However, it is important to understand what your child means by "eating healthier." Does your child plan to cut out junk food and eat more fruits and vegetables? Has your daughter decided to eat low-fat or non-fat foods only? Does your son eat significantly fewer calories than he did before? Is he constantly talking about food but rarely eats anything himself? Adolescents with eating disorders may exhibit any one or all of these behaviors.

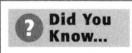

Did You Know...

• Dieting is one of the most important predictors of the development of an eating disorder.

• Females who diet seriously during adolescence are almost 20 times more likely to develop an eating disorder than those who do not diet.

If your child has made any of these dietary changes, you should monitor the corresponding behavior closely. Consider consulting a dietitian to help educate your child and provide you with guidance. If the behavior becomes extreme, consult your doctor.

Skipping Meals

The day-to-day pace for adolescents and their families in our culture is fast. Many teens are busy with school, socializing with their friends, taking part in sports, and working part-time. This often means eating on the run or skipping meals. Healthy teenagers will often eat at other times during the day to make up for these skipped meals. They will eat a large snack when they come home from school or frequently snack on food throughout the day.

However, young people with eating disorders often reduce their meal size significantly or skip meals altogether. They may begin by skipping breakfast or lunch, meals that often have little or no parental or adult supervision. Skipping meals is one of the first signs of an adolescent attempting to restrict food intake. Keep an eye on your child and try to discourage this behavior. Eating together as a family on a regular basis not only means that you can observe your children eating but also provides important family time.

Q: Is skipping breakfast an abnormal eating behavior for my son or is he just too busy to sit down to have a good meal?

A: More than 50% of adolescents (and a significant number of adults) do not eat breakfast. This in itself is not an indication that your son has an eating disorder. However, you might be more concerned if this is associated with a sudden change from his usual eating behavior and if he does not appear to be compensating by eating more throughout the rest of the day. If your son states that he is too rushed in the morning (as is often the case), then work with him to ensure that there are portable items he can take with him in the morning, such as juice boxes, small cartons of milk, granola or breakfast bars, and fruit.

Counting and Measuring

Often adolescents with an eating disorder are obsessed with reading food labels, looking for the number of calories or grams of fat that various foods contain, or weighing and measuring food portions. They will shift from eating food that they feel is 'fat food' or 'calorie dense' to 'safe' foods (foods the adolescent feels comfortable eating and are perceived to be less 'fattening' or less 'caloric'). Regardless of how hungry they may be, they dread the thought of eating any type of food that may be fattening. Thoughts about food can become constant and overwhelming. If your child is obsessed with counting and measuring, consult with a health-care professional.

Unusual Eating Practices

In their desperate effort to be thin, young people with eating disorders avoid foods with the necessary nutrition to maintain a healthy weight. To do so, they engage in unusual eating behaviors, pushing food around the plate, cutting food into small pieces, disposing pieces of food in a table napkin, chewing food and spitting it out before swallowing, getting up and down from the dinner table (thinking they will burn more calories), repeatedly standing at the dinner table (again, thinking that will burn more calories), and telling their parents that they have already eaten dinner when, in fact, they have not.

Adolescents with eating disorders tend to eat the same foods at the same time every day. They may begin to purchase 'diet' foods, such as low-fat shakes, low-fat dinners, or low-fat candy bars. Some may suddenly announce they have become vegetarian without any good stated reason.

Adolescents with eating disorders may have eating patterns that involve 'rules' about food. For example, they may only eat foods that are the same color or foods that have not touched other foods on their plate. Some adolescents may be so desperate to avoid eating any food that they hide it in various places, for example, in their night table, in a clothes cupboard, under their bed, or in a backpack.

They may also feel the need to get rid of food that they have eaten and want to purge. Be suspicious if your son or daughter regularly disappears to the washroom after meals. They could be vomiting or disposing of hidden food in the

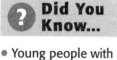
Did You Know...

• Young people with an eating disorder often avoid foods they once enjoyed and show disgust for them.

toilet or wastepaper basket. These are all very serious behaviors and indicate that your child may already have an eating disorder. You should be concerned. Talk to your daughter or son and let them know you are worried. Consult your doctor as soon as possible.

CASE STUDY Susan

At the request of her parents, Susan was discharged from the Eating Disorder Unit. Her parents felt that she could do just as well as an outpatient. They were committed to having her followed in the Outpatient Eating Disorder Clinic. One week after her hospitalization, she came for a clinic visit. She had gained weight and everyone celebrated. Over the next few weeks, things seemed to be okay. Susan got back to her life and continued to gain weight slowly.

During one of her clinic appointments, the doctor asked to speak to Susan's mother. The doctor had discovered some hidden coins taped to Susan's belly. Susan used these coins to make it look like she gained weight. When Susan was re-weighed without the coins, it became clear that she had not gained any weight since her discharge. In fact, she weighed less now than she did when she was discharged from the hospital. How did this happen?

Susan was crying when her mother came into the examination room. She admitted to cheating. She still denied that she had an eating disorder and only used the coins to make everyone happy that she had gained weight. Gaining weight was hard. She swore that she was doing everything she was supposed to be doing. She couldn't understand why she wasn't gaining weight.

Susan's mother was beginning to accept that her daughter had anorexia nervosa. How could she have missed the signs? Over the past few months, Susan had been cutting her food into tiny pieces and moving it around her plate, getting very upset if the family decided to go out for dinner, preparing all her own meals, eating all low-fat or no-fat foods, being very rigid about her exercise regimen, and spending lots of time on her own. Susan's father still couldn't see it. He insisted that his wife was overreacting.

Over the next few weeks, Susan's weight slowly went down and her parents both became more frustrated. Why couldn't she just eat and gain the weight?

The treatment team suggested another admission. Susan begged not to be admitted. She promised she would do anything to stay out of the hospital. Her social life and her schoolwork were going well. These would both suffer if her parents made her go into the hospital. Her parents knew she was right about this. They hoped that her friends and schoolwork were enough of a reason to get better. They agreed to make a deal with their daughter. She could stay out — if she gained an agreed upon amount of weight over the next month.

continued on page 86

Eating Alone

Young people with an eating disorder will often isolate themselves from others, especially around mealtime. This is particularly true when they realize that people have begun to notice that they are not eating normally. To avoid being found out by friends and family, adolescents may also claim that they have already eaten or report that they are not hungry.

You should be concerned that your daughter or son may have an eating disorder if you rarely see them eat or if they continuously make excuses about why they can't eat with you or other members of your family. For instance, excuses like "I ate already," "I ate at my friend's house," "I had a big lunch, so I'm not hungry for dinner," or "I'll get something later" are not uncommon among those suffering from an eating disorder and should raise concern.

Preoccupation with Food-Related Activities

Adolescents with eating disorders often develop a preoccupation with food-related activities, such as cooking and baking for others, reading cookbooks, downloading recipes off the Internet, or watching cooking shows on television. They will often prepare food (cakes, cookies, full-course meals) for family members but refuse to eat any themselves. They often claim they are no longer hungry or that they ate while preparing the food. This type of behavior may be a warning sign that your child has an eating disorder.

Binge Eating

Some adolescents with an eating disorder will binge, eating a large amount of food in 2 hours or less (for example, a gallon or 4-litre container of ice cream, two meat and cheese sandwiches, a big bag of chips, a box of cookies, and then a litre or quart of some beverage).

Binging may be triggered by the way adolescents feel about themselves or about a particular situation in their life. During this binge episode, they feel out of control, and after the episode, they feel depressed, humiliated, or guilty.

The binge may then be followed by a purge as they try to get rid of the food. Purging may involve self-induced vomiting or using laxatives and diuretics (water pills). Less immediate purging behavior includes drinking caffeine beverages

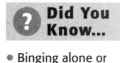

Did You Know...

● Binging alone or binging followed by purging is usually done "behind closed doors" or when other household members are not around.

● Commonly, adolescents will binge or binge and purge after school or in the middle of the night when everyone else is asleep.

to try to lose weight, taking diet pills, taking syrup of ipecac to induce vomiting, taking herbal remedies for weight loss, exercising to 'burn' calories, or fasting for a day or more.

Parents often find that they have food missing from the kitchen or need to buy larger amounts of food when they go to the grocery store. At the same time, they also notice that their child may be spending more time alone in the bedroom. Parents may notice numerous empty containers of food in the child's room or the garbage. Young people with this eating disorder may be so desperate to binge that they will steal money to buy the foods they crave to binge on.

CASE STUDY Jessica

Everyone notices when I gain weight. They start to joke about how I am just like my father. My mother has a small build and has always been thin…she eats like a bird. My father is the exact opposite. My parents love each other and joke about how opposites attract. They joke about how my brother takes after my mother and I take after my father.

No fair, why did I get my father's genes? I don't want to be fat. I hate the binging, but I can't stop it. I try to throw it up, but somehow I can never get it to work. I tried laxatives. Laxatives don't work…I never lose weight. So, I stopped buying them. They were expensive after all. I finally asked my parents for help and they took me to a diet doctor to help me lose weight. During the day, I followed the diet, and at night, I binged. I thought if I lost some weight, I would feel better about myself and stop binging. It didn't work.

continued on page 134

Bathroom Habits after Meals

Some young people with eating disorders will routinely excuse themselves from the table when they have completed eating their meal and immediately go to the bathroom. This may be in an attempt to get rid of the food they have eaten by vomiting. Often they will turn on the water taps to the sink or shower to conceal any sounds of vomiting.

Repeated and frequent vomiting can be life threatening. Consult your doctor if you have any worries about this.

Personal Behavior

The personal behavior of children or adolescents developing an eating disorder may also change. They may become dissatisfied with their physical appearance, exercise excessively, weigh themselves obsessively, become irritable, and have low self-esteem, among other problems.

Many children while developing an eating disorder are critical of their body shape, weight, and size. This behavior is especially telling when they believe that their body is fat, even though they are severely underweight. They may begin to talk obsessively about food and start to do things that are physically and emotionally dangerous to their health.

Frequent Weighing

Most healthy teenagers will weigh themselves occasionally as part of their natural interest in how they look. A person's weight normally fluctuates from day to day and throughout the day due to water intake, the amount of urine in their bladder, and food intake. These fluctuations are no cause for concern unless they are extreme.

However, if young people weigh themselves daily or more than once a day, be concerned, especially if the weight on the scale influences how your child feels. Teenagers with eating disorders often become distressed before and after weighing themselves.

Excessive Exercise

Adolescents with eating disorders may also exercise excessively and compulsively. In the beginning, this may appear to be quite normal, but soon it can interfere with other activities in their lives.

Some adolescents may become so obsessed with exercising that they will get upset or anxious if they have to miss an opportunity to work out. Often they will exercise in their rooms behind closed doors where they can't be seen or secretly exercise when household members have gone to sleep. They may run on the spot, jump rope, and do sit-ups and push-ups when no one is around to find out.

Some adolescents with eating disorders are involved in competitive sports that require enormous amounts of time and energy. This type of activity requires the young athlete to eat more in order to keep up with the increased energy demands. A teenager who does not meet energy requirements

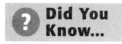
Did You Know...

• Some teenagers will engage in behaviors that they believe will help them burn calories: they may stand to do their homework, continually walk around while eating, or repetitively move their legs while sitting.

may become medically unwell in a relatively short period of time, putting them at risk of severe medical problems, including death. An informed health-care professional, coach, or teacher should be involved to ensure that participation in these sports or activities is done in a healthy and safe way.

If you are concerned that your child is exercising too much, then you should consult your doctor. Your doctor will help you understand whether this behavior is excessive. Your doctor can also provide you and your child with clear guidelines about how much exercise is appropriate and how much food your child should eat to stay healthy.

> **Q:** My 13-year-old daughter is exercising in her room for 2 to 3 hours every day. Should I be worried?
>
> **A:** It is ideal for children and adolescents to have some physical activity incorporated in their daily activity, but this exercise should be social, fun, and moderate in nature. When kids begin to indulge in extreme, secretive, or solitary exercise, then parents should be concerned. The goals of this type of exercise may be unhealthy.

Irritability and Mood Swings

Parents of adolescents developing an eating disorder often comment that their child is undergoing a change in personality. They often become irritable or upset about things that normally wouldn't bother them. Some parents notice that their children become very depressed and withdrawn.

Distorted Body Image and Low Self-Esteem

Healthy adolescents naturally care about how other people see them, and it is not uncommon for them to have occasional negative thoughts about who they are and how they look. Teenagers with eating disorders, however, are often consumed with the way they look. They develop a distorted body image. For instance, a girl with anorexia nervosa thinks she is 'fat' even when she is underweight.

Self-esteem involves how people like and value themselves. Young people with positive self-esteem are able to feel good about who they are and appreciate their unique qualities. Adolescents with poor body image and self-esteem, however, have negative thoughts about themselves, such as, "I'm ugly," "I'm fat," or "I'm stupid."

Parents can play an important role in identifying when their children are not feeling good about themselves. Parents

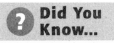

Did You Know...

● Sometimes poor body image and low self-esteem are very difficult for adolescents to handle on their own.

● Some young people with an eating disorder may become depressed, lose interest in their friends, use drugs or alcohol, restrict their food intake, or binge and purge.

can help their children by talking about these feelings. Other times parents may need to get help from health-care professionals, especially if these feelings are affecting your child's ability to function normally.

Q: My 14-year-old daughter says she's too fat and wants to diet. I think she looks fine. What should I do?

A: Teenagers who are concerned about their weight should see their doctor before considering dietary changes. Many normal-weight adolescent girls have unrealistic ideas about how their bodies should look.

In general, diets are not recommended for growing children. Unsupervised dieting can jeopardize a child's intake of calories, vitamins, minerals, and other nutrients needed for proper development. Moderation in food intake and physical activity can improve your child's sense of well-being.

Parents can also help teens by being good role models. Children are more likely to eat right and exercise regularly if their parents do, too.

Inflexibility

Often parents notice that their child has become increasingly inflexible. The child may express great distress, anxiety, or anger at changes to routine. This may be a sign of an eating disorder. Adolescents with eating disorders are always planning ahead about when they are going to eat, what they are going to eat, and when, where, and if they are going to purge. If this plan is changed, it can cause a great deal of distress or anxiety for the teenager. Parents can help their children become more flexible, by talking to them and helping them come up with solutions. If this behavior is part of an established eating disorder, you may need professional help to deal with it.

Medical Excuses

Some teenagers attempt to explain their weight loss or eating behaviors as being due to medical illness. They may report feeling nauseous or vomiting due to stomach pains. They may repeatedly tell you that they are not feeling well. Consider taking your child to your doctor who may do a workup for a medical problem that can cause these signs and symptoms. It is not unusual for a young person with an eating disorder to be evaluated by a doctor for nausea, vomiting, stomach pains, and constipation before finally being diagnosed with an eating disorder.

COMMON SIGNS AND SYMPTOMS OF EATING DISORDERS

Parents can assist their children and health-care professionals by being alert to changes in physical appearance, eating behavior, personal behavior, and social behavior that may indicate the development of an eating disorder. Take a moment to check off the changes in appearance and behavior listed below that your child may be undergoing. Discuss these changes with your child, and seek medical advice if you are still concerned.

Physical Appearance

- ☐ Weight loss, fluctuation
- ☐ Failure to gain weight or height normally
- ☐ Delay in the onset of puberty
- ☐ Loss of menstrual period
- ☐ Irregular menstrual periods
- ☐ Yellow-tinged skin
- ☐ Thinning hair/hair loss
- ☐ Fine downy hair, known as lanugo hair
- ☐ Conjunctival hemorrhages
- ☐ Swollen glands (chipmunk cheeks)
- ☐ Calluses or scars on the back of hands
- ☐ Dental caries (cavities)

Eating Behaviors

- ☐ Dieting
- ☐ Changes in types of food eaten
- ☐ Skipping meals
- ☐ Counting calories and grams of fat
- ☐ Weighing or measuring food
- ☐ Unusual eating practices
- ☐ Food rules
- ☐ Disgust for previously favorite foods
- ☐ Eating alone
- ☐ Increased interest in all things to do with food

- ☐ Binging and hoarding food
- ☐ Spending time in the bathroom immediately after meals
- ☐ Vomiting or purging after meals
- ☐ Use of laxatives, diet pills, diuretics, ipecac, herbal remedies
- ☐ Use of excessive caffeine

Personal Behavior

- ☐ Frequent weighing
- ☐ Excessive exercise
- ☐ New interest in competitive sports
- ☐ Anxiety at missing routine exercise
- ☐ Extreme concern with appearance
- ☐ Distorted body image
- ☐ Wearing baggy clothes
- ☐ Low self-esteem
- ☐ Inflexibility and resistance to change
- ☐ Irritability, mood swings, 'personality change'
- ☐ Medical excuses for behavior

Social Behavior

- ☐ Spending more time alone
- ☐ Increasing social isolation from old friends
- ☐ Poor concentration, attention span
- ☐ Decreased school performance
- ☐ Stealing (food or money to buy food)

WORKSHEET

EATING DISORDERED BEHAVIORS, THOUGHTS, AND FEELINGS

This checklist of behaviors, thoughts, and feelings that children and adolescents can experience while beginning to struggle with an eating disorder might help you to recognize whether your child is developing an eating disorder. These behaviors, thoughts, and feelings are not normal or healthy.

Check those items that apply to your child and family. The more items you check, the more concerning your child's problem may be. The intensity and duration of each risk factor can influence the seriousness of your child's problem. This checklist will allow you to document your concerns and discuss them with your child together with your family doctor or pediatrician.

Keep in mind that just because your child may be experiencing one or more of these factors does not necessarily mean that your child has or is developing an eating disorder.

☐ My daughter continually makes comments like "I'm so fat" or "I want to be thinner than my friends."

☐ My son gets very anxious, angry, or upset if he can't exercise.

☐ My daughter had regular menstrual periods for 2 years, but she hasn't had a menstrual period for the last 4 months.

☐ My daughter is constantly talking about what she is going to prepare for her next meal.

☐ My son insists on coming grocery shopping with me. He is adamant about buying all "no fat" foods.

☐ My son refuses to go out to restaurants with our family. He always complains that there is nothing healthy for him to eat.

☐ Our son never eats with the family or his friends. He almost always chooses to eat by himself.

☐ My daughter has been cooking meals and baking all kinds of desserts for the family. But we never see her eat any of it.

☐ Whenever I come home from work, my daughter informs me that she has already eaten her dinner. She rarely has dinner with us anymore.

☐ My daughter gets very upset and agitated if her meal schedule is changed in anyway.

☐ My son eats the same food at each meal every day. There is absolutely no variety in types of food or time. He is completely rigid about his meals.

☐ My daughter thinks if she were thinner, she would be happier.

☐ My daughter reads recipes, cookbooks, calorie charts, and books about dieting and exercise.

☐ My daughter used to love to have sleepovers with her friends. Now she refuses to go over to any of her friends' homes or have them at our home.

☐ My son is very sad and irritable.

☐ My child feels guilty when she eats.

☐ I had anorexia nervosa as an adolescent and am now totally recovered.

WORKSHEET

- ☐ My daughter spends a lot of time on her own. She never sees her friends anymore.

- ☐ The day after I go grocery shopping, I'm missing a lot of food from the kitchen cupboard and fridge.

- ☐ My daughter does unusual things to her food, cutting it into tiny pieces and moving it around her plate. I have even seen her hide her food in her napkin and feed it to our dog.

- ☐ My son is never happy who he is or what he acc

- ☐ My daughter always asks to table immediately after she h___ ___ er meal to go to the bathroom. Sne is spending a long time in the bathroom.

- ☐ My son was caught stealing food from our grocery store.

- ☐ My daughter is a figure skater and informed us that ever since she lost some weight, her performance has improved.

Social Behavior

There are a number of changes in social behavior that are a part of normal adolescent development. These include increased focus on appearance, increased independence from family, more time spent with peers, and increased sensitivity to comments from parents and others. When adolescents withdraw from many of their usual activities with peers and family, this can indicate a number of potential problems, including depression, alcohol or substance abuse, or eating disorders. If you have concerns that your child is having problems with any of these issues, you should discuss them with your doctor.

Spending More Time Alone

Children and adolescents with eating disorders are likely to miss out on many activities of daily living. The eating disorder causes them to be detached from different social activities, especially if the activities are food related. They can't go over to a friend's house for dinner, can't go to birthday parties, and can't have Christmas brunch at grandmother's house. These adolescents seem to withdraw into themselves, staying away from family and friends. Over time, parents often report that their children spend increasing amounts of time alone. They don't participate in social activities with their friends any longer.

Much of their time is spent planning the next meal, calculating how they will burn off calories, and worrying about how they can avoid uncomfortable social situations that involve food and eating. Sometimes, the adolescent becomes depressed, sad, and lonely and may not feel worthy of friends.

Take this behavior seriously. Do not assume this is a phase your child is going through.

Q: My son used to be very busy on the weekends with his friends. Recently, he has been spending an awful lot of time on his own. He has been focused on his appearance, his schoolwork, and cooking for our family. This is so unlike him. Should we be doing anything?

A: Normal adolescent development includes a number of changes in social behavior, such as focus on appearance, increased independence from family, more time spent with peers, and increased sensitivity to comments from parents and others. However, if your son has had a major change in his interests, a change in his grades at school, or withdraws from his peers and family, this may indicate that your child is having some difficulties.

There are a number of problems that can present like this, including depression, substance abuse, or eating disorders. If you have concerns, discuss them with your doctor.

Poor Attention Span, Change in School Performance

Adolescents with eating disorders may have more difficulty concentrating and focusing on schoolwork and other tasks of daily living. School performance may be affected. However, adolescents with eating disorders are often extraordinary at concealing these difficulties. In fact, parents and teachers are shocked to learn that this may be one of the complications of an eating disorder since the young person is so 'high-functioning.'

Adolescents may spend more time doing homework so that they can achieve the same grades because their concentration has been affected by their starved condition.

What Is a Parent To Do?

If you are concerned about changes in your children's physical appearance, eating behaviors, or moods and feelings, find out more about their feelings and thoughts. Ask them what is bothering them.

Parents are sometimes worried about how their child will react when asking these questions. They fear their child will be upset or angry with them. When speaking to your children about their health and safety, do so in a sensitive, calm, and concerned way. Focus on behaviors that you have witnessed, describe them, and express your resulting feelings. Try using "I feel" statements.

Chances are your child is probably very frightened about these behaviors as well. However, young people with eating disorders may be initially defensive, unwilling to admit or perhaps even recognize they have a problem. They may even vociferously deny that they have an eating problem. Alternatively, they may welcome your concern and ask for help. They may have been waiting for you to respond, consciously or unconsciously.

If you have concern that your children are showing physical signs of an eating disorder, or if they are behaving in a way that makes you wonder about whether they have an eating disorder, you should approach your family doctor or pediatrician for an evaluation. If your child had a cough that wasn't getting any better, you would do the same thing...that is, you would tell your child you are concerned about the cough and it was time to go to the doctor.

SAMPLE "I FEEL" STATEMENTS

"I feel" statements can help avoid situations where your child feels judged. This will help reduce defensive behaviors that commonly arise when these difficult topics are broached by family members.

"When I see how much weight you have lost, I feel very worried about your health. I'm frightened that you have a serious problem. What happens to you is very important to me."

"I see that your eating has changed lately. You seem to be eating a lot when you come home from school and spending a lot of time in the bathroom afterward. I'm worried that you are binging and throwing up. I'm worried because this can be dangerous to your health. This can be embarrassing to talk about, but I want you to know that I am here to help and not to judge."

"Your friends have been calling and wanting you to go out with them, but you keep turning them down. I'm worried about this because you've always enjoyed spending time with them. I can't help think that there is something wrong. Can we talk about it?"

"I've noticed that you have been leaving food on your plate every night at dinner. You seem to be cutting your food into tiny pieces. I was most concerned when you fed the dog the food on your plate. When I see this happening night after night, I worry that you're trying to lose weight in a way that's not healthy."

CHAPTER 7

What Are the Possible Medical Complications of Eating Disorders?

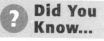
Most people do not realize the extent to which eating disorders can be harmful to the physical health of children and adolescents for a number of reasons. For one, many of these possible health problems are 'silent' and not detectable simply by looking at a person. The body is also remarkably good at adjusting to the malnourished state, to the extent that a person with an eating disorder may 'feel fine' even though the internal organs are not working properly. However well-disguised, these problems can be severe. Eating disorders can cause death.

Some medical complications of eating disorders require immediate admission to hospital — examples include extremely low body weight, very low heart rate, low blood pressure, low body temperature, irregular heart rhythms (arrhythmias), and electrolyte abnormalities. Other problems may not be an immediate threat to a child or adolescent's health, but may put them at risk for long-term health concerns — low bone density, failure to attain ultimate adult height, and absence of menstrual periods, for example. Health problems that are not life threatening may still affect a young person's health for years to come.

Doctors and nurses who care for children and adolescents with eating disorders, as well as parents and other caregivers, need to monitor these young people carefully for the development of physical problems. Depending on the nature or severity of the problem, this monitoring may require frequent visits to a clinic or may even require admission to hospital.

Many parents are overwhelmed by the long list of problems that their children may experience as a consequence of their eating disorder. The good news is that many of these problems can be treated. The majority of children and adolescents with eating disorders will do well with appropriate treatment.

INDICATIONS FOR ADMISSION TO HOSPITAL

If the medical complications of the eating disorder are serious, your child may need to be admitted to hospital for treatment. Hospitalization will allow for safe and adequate weight gain, medical and/or psychiatric stabilization, the initiation of safe and healthy eating habits, and ultimately a better outcome for the affected child. This list of symptoms is modified from The Society for Adolescent Medicine Guidelines (December 2003).

- Weight loss has been severe or rapid
- Dehydration
- Electrolyte disturbances
- Irregular heart rhythms (arrhythmias)
- Low blood pressure
- Extremely low heart rate
- Low body temperature
- Arrested growth and development

- Failure of outpatient or day-hospital treatment
- Acute food refusal
- Uncontrollable binging and/or purging
- Fainting/seizures/confusion/heart failure
- Psychiatric emergencies, such as suicidal thoughts or severe depression, that interfere with the treatment of the eating disorder

Low Body Weight and Starvation

Although not a feature of all types of eating disorders, low body weight is a characteristic of anorexia nervosa, as well as some other types of eating disorders. In addition to being underweight, people develop an abnormal body composition as a result of being undernourished.

Normally, the body is composed of a certain amount of fat, muscle, bone, and fluid. After not eating enough for a long enough period of time, the body starts to feed on itself for energy. At this point, the body is in a state of starvation. This results in significant decreases in fat and muscle stores.

Society seems to have become increasingly 'fat-phobic' over the past few years. The prevailing messages suggest that the less body fat you have, the better off you are. Not so! The truth is that each component of our bodies (including fat) serves a vital function. Without enough fat, our bodies do not work the way they should.

Besides helping to keep us warm and padding our bones for protection, body fat is one of the crucial factors allowing young women to have regular menstrual periods. This is why underweight people are at risk of low body temperatures, pressure sores over areas where the bones are not covered by anything but skin, and loss of regular menstrual periods.

In addition to the ill health effects of abnormal body composition, low body weight by itself can be dangerous. In a starved state, the body decides to use the tiny amounts of energy that it is receiving very efficiently. Essentially, the body goes into slow-mode. Everything seems to move at a slower pace — brain function, heart rate, body temperature, and movements of the stomach and intestines. For this reason, health-care professionals who assess and treat severely underweight children or adolescents with eating disorders would likely suggest admission to hospital for slow weight restoration and close medical monitoring as the first line of treatment.

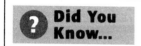

Did You Know...

• Severely underweight people are at risk of sudden collapse and death.

Brain Changes

There are changes in the various brain tissues of malnourished adolescents with eating disorders. Brain scans of children and adolescents with anorexia nervosa have shown that parts of the brain undergo structural changes during the starved state. Some of these changes return to normal after weight gain, but there is evidence that some damage may be permanent. The impact of these changes on brain structure is unknown.

Besides changes in brain structure, studies have also shown alterations in the way the brain works. These changes in brain structure and function may explain some of the symptoms that adolescents with eating disorders report and that health-care professionals observe — concentration difficulties, mood changes, and changes in the way people understand information. One's ability to think logically or understand abstract information may be affected. In spite of maintaining high marks at school, some children and adolescents with eating disorders will admit that it takes them much longer to do homework than it did prior to the weight loss.

Heart, Blood Pressure, and Circulation Problems

Eating disorders can affect the heart in many ways. Some heart abnormalities can be detected by physical exam (checking the pulse and blood pressure and listening to the heart). Other problems require specialized testing, such as an electrocardiogram (EKG) or echocardiogram.

Low blood pressures can also be observed in children and adolescents with eating disorders. Irregular heart rhythms (arrhythmias) may be caused by low body weight or abnormal minerals in the blood. All of these abnormalities are potentially life threatening. If one or more of these abnormalities is present, admission to hospital for close medical monitoring would be required.

Treatment consists of weight restoration in a hospital. An intravenous solution containing glucose, minerals, and water fed into the body through a vein may be required for extremely low blood pressure. Supplements of certain additional minerals may be required, depending on the levels in the blood.

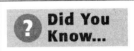
Did You Know...

- The most common heart abnormality observed in underweight adolescents with eating disorders is a very slow heart rate — also called bradycardia.

- Bradycardia is potentially life threatening.

ELECTROCARDIOGRAM (EKG)

An EKG (also known as an ECG) is a relatively simple test that requires the placement of a number of leads (stickers) over the body. A few stickers are placed on the chest, the arms, and the legs. The stickers measure the electrical activity of the heart and produce a print-out for the doctors to review. This print-out is called an EKG. Doctors use the EKG to look for heart disease or abnormal rhythms (arrhythmias). There are well-established normal values for the various measurements that can be obtained from an EKG. It takes only a few minutes to do the test and get results.

ECHOCARDIOGRAM

An echocardiogram is a test that uses ultrasound (sound waves) to produce a picture of the heart. Important information about the valves of the heart and the function of the muscles of the heart can be obtained. This test requires the expertise of health-care professionals who are specially trained to do the test and to interpret the results. For this reason, it may take some time before the results of this test are available. This test is painless, requiring a patient to lie still while a special instrument is placed next to the chest.

Another potential life-threatening complication found in children and adolescents with eating disorders is heart failure. Heart failure is a condition that causes the heart to pump blood less effectively than normal. As a result, fluid can collect in the lungs and other parts of the body. Fortunately, this happens rarely.

The structure of the heart can also become abnormal in malnutrition. Just as the muscles of the body become smaller with excessive weight loss, the heart muscle can also become smaller. In fact, medical research has shown that the hearts of underweight people with anorexia nervosa have thinner walls than normal.

The low heart rate seen in underweight adolescents with eating disorders is very different from the low heart rate observed in well-trained athletes. Well-trained athletes have a normal amount of heart muscle and their hearts work more efficiently during exercise. The hearts of underweight people with anorexia nervosa have thinner walls and often do not react appropriately to exercise.

Circulation problems are very common in adolescents with eating disorders. The hands and feet may become cold and may also develop a bluish discoloration. Many parents comment that their child's hands and feet have become "ice-cold."

Electrolyte Abnormalities

Electrolytes can be deranged in adolescents with eating disorders. Recurrent vomiting puts people at risk for developing low potassium in the blood and arrhythmias that can result in death. Some people with eating disorders will drink excess amounts of fluids in order to give a false impression of weight gain. This is a risky behavior because excessive intake of water can result in an extremely low sodium level in the blood. The consequences of an extremely low sodium level include confusion, seizures, coma, and death.

Fortunately, many of these mineral abnormalities can be detected in the blood work of adolescents with eating disorders and treated with supplements by mouth or by intravenous. Depending on the mineral level, treatment may occur in an outpatient or in an inpatient setting.

Once a person has been starving for a period of time and is then re-fed, there can be changes in some of the minerals in

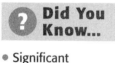
Did You Know...

• Significant abnormalities in minerals in the blood (electrolytes) may result in arrhythmias, muscle weakness, cramps, confusion, seizures, coma, and death.

• Common electrolyte abnormalities include low potassium, low or high sodium, low phosphorous, and low calcium.

the blood. This is part of the reason why the initial part of re-feeding and slow weight restoration should happen in hospital where there can be careful and constant medical monitoring. Blood work will often be monitored daily for the first few days after admission to hospital.

Body Temperature Control

A common finding among people who have lost significant amounts of weight is a low body temperature. You may see that undernourished people have a low body temperature or they are unable to maintain a normal body temperature when exposed to cool surrounding temperatures. Affected people often report that they feel cold when everyone else is fine or that they have to wear many layers of clothes in order to keep themselves warm.

Body temperature is regulated by a part of the brain called the hypothalamus. The hypothalamus may also be affected by malnutrition.

Digestive System Problems

As a result of the intestines slowing down, many adolescents with eating disorders experience constipation (hard, dry stools that are difficult to pass) due to their excessive weight loss. Other factors that may aggravate constipation include inadequate intake of fiber-containing foods, as well as inadequate intake of fluids.

Besides constipation, adolescents with eating disorders may experience bloating of their stomachs after meals. They may complain of feeling over full or nauseated. This is not an uncommon feeling once a person has been starving for a period of time and begins to eat larger volumes of food. These symptoms go away as the body adjusts to eating larger quantities of food. Besides restoration of normal nutrition, there is no specific treatment indicated (sometimes smaller, more frequent meals may provide some relief). Adolescents with eating disorders should be reassured that these symptoms will go away over time as they continue to eat properly.

TREATMENT FOR CONSTIPATION

The standard treatment of constipation in adolescents with eating disorders is:

1. Restore normal weight.

2. Supply adequate amount of nutrition and fluids (ensuring enough fiber content).

3. Add extra fiber to the diet.

Stool softeners or laxatives may be prescribed if the constipation is severe. These medications are rarely needed and should not be used without specific recommendations from a health-care professional.

Kidney Problems

The kidney has many important roles — to ensure a normal balance of fluid within the body, to maintain a normal blood pressure, to get rid of waste, and to maintain normal levels of certain minerals in the blood. In addition to restricting their intake of food, some adolescents with eating disorders also restrict their intake of fluid. Children and adolescents with eating disorders may also induce vomiting, abuse laxatives or diuretics, or use diet pills. Unfortunately, these behaviors can lead to serious medical problems.

Kidney failure refers to a situation where the kidneys stop functioning properly. This can lead to a buildup of waste materials in the blood, high blood pressure, an abnormal buildup of fluid within the body, and abnormal electrolytes (minerals in the blood). In the case of mild kidney dysfunction, intravenous fluids may be the only required treatment. In more serious cases, more intensive treatments may be required, including dialysis. Dialysis is a mechanical process that partly performs the work that healthy kidneys normally do. The main function of dialysis is clearing wastes from the blood. Monitoring in an intensive care unit may also be required.

There are additional actions that can potentially be harmful to the kidneys. An example is ingesting excessive amounts of protein (in the form of nutritional supplements). There are reports in the medical literature of kidney dysfunction associated with use of protein supplements, such as creatine.

? Did You Know...

• Excessive restriction of fluid, frequent vomiting, laxative abuse, or diuretic abuse can lead to dehydration, low blood pressure, abnormal electrolytes, and, rarely, kidney failure.

Bone Problems

Bone development starts in the womb and continues throughout childhood, adolescence, and early adulthood. Bones continue to be built and strengthened throughout these phases of life. Adolescence is the time when maximal bone is laid down. By late adolescence to early adulthood, individuals have attained their peak bone mass (or achieved maximum bone strength). After the early thirties, bones gradually become less dense and strong over the rest of an adult's life. Bone loss is accelerated in post-menopausal women due to low levels of estrogen.

Low bone density is a frequent, early, and common complication of children and adolescents with anorexia nervosa. Osteoporosis is a term used to describe bones that are significantly less dense than normal. The bones are more fragile than normal and thus more susceptible to fractures. The problems associated with low bone density (e.g., bone fractures) may not show themselves during childhood or adolescence.

The best way to measure a young person's bone density is by a test called dual energy X-ray absorptiometry, also commonly referred to as DEXA. This is a painless scan that measures the bone density of the hip, spine, and whole body.

The best treatment for osteoporosis is weight restoration and ensuring adequate amounts of calcium and vitamin D in the diet. So far, hormonal treatment, such as estrogen, has not been shown to be beneficial. This area continues to be studied.

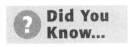

? Did You Know...

- Even with treatment, it is not known whether or not the deficits in bone density found in children and adolescents with anorexia nervosa are completely reversible.

MAKING STRONG BONES

There are several important factors that help to make bones strong and to keep them that way:

- Normal body weight

- Adequate calcium intake

- Adequate vitamin D intake

- Sex hormones — estrogen in females and testosterone in males

- Moderate amounts of carefully monitored weight-bearing exercise. Weight-bearing exercise includes any activity where your feet and legs carry your own weight. This includes such activities as walking and dancing, as well as team sports like soccer, basketball, or field hockey.

CASE STUDY Susan

Susan and her parents got the bad news at her next appointment. Her doctor had recommended that her bone mineral density be tested and it was found to be abnormally low. The doctor explained that girls with anorexia nervosa often have low bone mineral density. This condition is concerning since the bones are more fragile than normal and, therefore, more susceptible to fractures. Her parents were shocked…this didn't happen to adolescent girls. Susan's grandmother had osteoporosis and required a hip replacement after a fall.

The doctor informed Susan and her parents that weight gain helped to increase bone mineral density. In addition, the doctor recommended that Susan should have at least 1500 mg of calcium in her diet and take 400 IU of vitamin D. Adolescence is a crucial time for young girls to "lay down" bone and the doctors wanted to make sure that Susan, with the support of her parents, did everything possible to ensure this.

Susan's mother and *now* her father were really worried, but not Susan. She thought everyone was overreacting. No problem… she would take the calcium and the vitamin D. The doctors were making a big deal out of nothing…once again!

The eating disorder team reminded Susan's parents that teenagers often feel invincible. What were they going to do?

continued on page 167

Menstrual Changes

Erratic eating, extreme fasting, purging behaviors, dieting, changes in mood, and significant weight loss can all interfere with the normal menstrual cycle. The result of these abnormal eating behaviors is irregular or absent menstrual periods.

The absence of menstrual periods, called amenorrhea, is a classic feature of anorexia nervosa. Primary amenorrhea is seen in adolescents who have never had a menstrual period when they otherwise should have. Secondary amenorrhea occurs in adolescents who used to have regular menstrual periods but have stopped having them for more than 3 months. In fact, the hormone estrogen, which is an important female hormone responsible for the development of the breasts, the vagina, and the uterus, as well as the building up of the uterine lining before each menstrual period, is very low in adolescents with anorexia nervosa.

Estrogen has other important functions as well. It helps to maintain strong bones. Therefore, low levels of estrogen found in adolescents with anorexia nervosa puts them at risk for having low bone density and, therefore, brittle bones.

The treatment of amenorrhea is weight restoration and elimination of chaotic eating patterns. For most adolescents, it will take several months after attaining a normal weight before normal menstrual periods resume. It is not uncommon to have irregular bleeding or spotting during the recovery phase of an eating disorder. Periods will normalize over time with sustained treatment. Rarely, adolescents will continue to have menstrual periods or have their menstrual periods return when they are underweight. It is important to remember that menstrual periods are not the only measure of health.

Treatment with an oral contraceptive pill (OCP) may restore regular menstrual bleeding, but it does not necessarily protect bones. Bleeding that occurs with OCP treatment does not necessarily mean a young woman is at a normal weight or has physically recovered from anorexia nervosa.

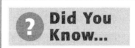

Did You Know...

• Doctors routinely check hormone levels of females who have eating disorders.

• The reproductive hormone levels of adolescents with an eating disorder are often similar to the hormone levels of children who have not yet reached puberty.

Growth Failure

One feature of eating disorders that is unique to children and adolescents is the impact that the eating disorder can have on growth and development. Until adulthood, one of the most important tools used to assess health is the pediatric growth curve. Normally, children make gains in both height and weight as they progress from infancy to adulthood. Adolescence is a time of rapid growth and development — the growth spurt occurs during this time until final adult height is achieved. In addition, the reproductive organs mature. Weight loss or failure to make the expected gains in weight and height generally indicates a serious health problem and is always a cause for concern.

If a child or adolescent is not taking in enough nutrition to gain weight, growth in height may suffer as well. There is a critical period during adolescence after which no further growth in height can occur. For this reason, some people with eating disorders may not only have a slow down in their growth as a result of malnutrition, they may also experience growth arrest. They may never attain their full adult height potential.

Teeth and Neck Problems

Significant damage to the teeth can occur from recurrent vomiting as a result of repeat contact of the teeth with stomach acids. In the case of repeated vomiting, young people may also develop enlarged salivary glands that can give the appearance of swollen jaws or cheeks. Neither of these conditions is life threatening but can have a significant impact on your child's quality of life.

Skin Abnormalities

Dry skin, with yellowish coloring of the palms and soles, is a common finding among children and adolescents with eating disorders. Another finding, usually seen in people who are significantly underweight, is lanugo hair — a fine, downy hair that can grow over the entire body, but often is seen most prominently over the back and neck. This usually goes away with weight restoration. If adolescents stick their fingers down their throat in an attempt to make themselves vomit, they may develop calluses (areas of hard skin) on the back of their hand, a condition known as Russell's sign. It will slowly resolve when this method of self-induced vomiting ceases.

Nutritional Deficiencies

Overt nutritional deficiencies are actually rarely seen in adolescents with eating disorders. Often, if a specific meal plan is being adhered to, there is no need for vitamins or supplements.

Death

There is an increased risk for early death among adolescents with eating disorders. Some of these deaths are related to medical complications and some are as a result of suicide. Eating disorders have the highest mortality rate of any psychiatric illness.

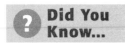

Did You Know...

• Because growth can only occur up until a certain point, the treatment of growth impairment in early adolescence is considered to be a relatively urgent situation.

• Restoration of a normal body weight to maximize potential for growth is the recommended treatment for this problem. Since time is of the essence, aggressive treatment in the form of admission to hospital may be indicated.

Recovery

Despite the possible fatal outcome of medical complications of eating disorders, most children and adolescents will recover with appropriate medical treatment and encouraging support from family and friends. Recovery is very seldom spontaneous, however. While weight restoration can occur over several weeks to months in hospital, the other aspects of an eating disorder (abnormal body image, fears of certain foods, fears of gaining weight) take much longer to improve.

Visiting the Emergency Department

At some point in your child's illness, you may need to take your son or daughter to your local Emergency Department for the assessment and treatment of an acute medical or psychiatric emergency resulting from their eating disorder. This could happen while your child is on a waiting list for treatment or is in treatment at an outpatient clinic or day hospital program. Regardless, children with eating disorders can present at anytime with serious medical and psychiatric emergencies. Food and fluid restriction or binging and purging can lead to a variety of serious and life-threatening medical and psychiatric problems.

Parent's Role in an Emergency Visit

Parent's naturally play a key role in any emergency visit, from simply transporting your child to the hospital to advocating for full attention from the staff.

If your child reveals an acute medical problem, has attempted suicide, or is threatening suicide, you need to take this situation seriously. Don't delay calling your doctor or taking your child to your nearest hospital emergency department.

It is not uncommon for children to protest adamantly a visit to the emergency department. Don't give in to their objections! Most parents are unable to assess the severity of an acute medical or psychiatric problem resulting from an eating disorder. Sometimes parents will take their child to their local emergency department because they are worried that there is something seriously wrong and it turns out to be

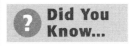

Did You Know...

● It can take 5 to 6 years before there is complete recovery from an eating disorder. For this reason, ongoing monitoring as an outpatient will be recommended by the treatment team.

● Some people may require more than one admission to hospital over the course of their illness.

a minor concern. Don't feel bad if this has happened to you… even if it's happened more than once! A parent's job is to advocate for the health and well-being of their child. The doctor's job is to make a diagnosis and determine the seriousness of the situation. If you think that your child has a medical or psychiatric emergency, get them immediate medical care.

The emergency department is often a busy and hectic place. You may have to ensure that your child's symptoms are taken seriously. If you and your child are in the emergency department for an extended period of time, then ongoing monitoring will be required. Talk to the staff about your child's nutritional and fluid needs. Discuss any abnormalities with the doctor in the emergency department and make sure the doctor explains the seriousness and the risks associated with these changes.

If the doctor sends you home, be sure you understand what kind of follow-up is necessary. Make sure you write everything down so that you can inform your health-care professional about the details of your visit to the emergency department.

EMERGENCY DEPARTMENT QUICK REFERENCE GUIDE

If you need to take your child to the emergency department, be sure to inform the staff about any previous or existing medical instability or psychiatric emergency. The staff will want to know what led you to bring your child to the emergency department. Expect to answer many questions about your child and be prepared for the following procedures.

History

- Known eating disorder (anorexia nervosa, bulimia nervosa, binge eating disorder, eating disorder not otherwise specified).
- Suspected eating disorders, such as food refusal, significant weight loss, severe malnutrition, dietary restriction, unusual eating behaviors, fear of fatness, distorted body image.
- History of weight loss (onset, maximum and minimum weights, rate of weight loss).
- History of self-induced vomiting, binging and purging, dieting, excessive exercise. Use of laxatives, diuretics, or ipecac. How often and last episode?
- History of ingestions (medications, weight loss aids, complementary and alternative medicine supplements, street drugs).

- Menstrual history. Reached menarche? Primary or secondary amenorrhea?
- Known or suspected psychiatric history, such as depression or obsessive compulsive disorder.
- Current or past history of self-harm, thoughts of suicide, or suicide attempt.
- Prior assessment and management of this condition (medical and psychiatric, inpatient, outpatient, health-care professional's name and location).
- Past psychiatric history and family psychiatric history.
- Last intake of food and fluids, and assessment of past 24-hour intake.

Physical Examination

- Height, weight and body mass index, and percentiles on growth curve for age (best done in a hospital gown without footwear).
- Bradycardia, orthostatic heart rate, and blood pressure changes, arrhythmia, oral temperature.
- Hydration status.
- Lanugo hair, Russell's sign (callus on dorsum of hand), parotid swelling and other scarring (evidence of self-harm).
- Dental erosion (may occur with chronic vomiting over several years).
- Signs of fluid overload (congestive heart failure, peripheral swelling of hands or feet).
- Mental status changes.

Laboratory Investigations

- 12-lead EKG
- Cardiac monitor if heart rate < 50 beats per minute or abnormal EKG.
- Urine dipstick with first void (pH and specific gravity).
- Complete blood count with differential, erythrocyte sedimentation rate, electrolytes (sodium, potassium, chloride), glucose, blood urea nitrogen, creatinine, calcium, phosphate, magnesium, venous blood gas, amylase, liver function tests.

Consultations and Referrals

The staff in the Emergency Department may want to consult the eating disorder experts in your local hospital (pediatricians, adolescent medicine specialists, and child and adolescent psychiatrists).

CHAPTER 8

What Is My Child Thinking?

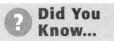 **Did You Know...**

• Eating disorders have the ability to make an adolescent, who is just skin and bones, feel 'fat', as if they are looking through a distorted circus mirror.

• They have the power to make your once highly sensitive child become dishonest, aggressive, and secretive.

Take a moment to recall the story of Snow White. This is a tale of a young, bright girl who is tricked by a Wicked Witch in disguise. Snow White is intrigued by the Wicked Witch when she comes to visit and eats the poisoned apple she is offered by her guest. A child or adolescent suffering with an eating disorder is in a similar situation as Snow White. Although the eating disorder is terribly harmful, the child welcomes the illness when it is offered. The intentions of the Wicked Witch, however destructive, are not recognized.

Why is this illness often welcomed? Why would a young person choose this lifestyle when the consequences are so frightening and horrible? Why does a teenager decide to give up her friends, her pleasant disposition, and her relationships within her own family? Why does the child shrug when he is presented with the knowledge that an eating disorder is a serious life threatening disease? How do we understand why a teenager would accept the discomfort of extreme hunger or choose to binge and purge?

In their confusion and despair, parents are left to exclaim, "Why don't you just eat?" or "Just stop throwing up!"

There is no doubt that eating disorders are not only confusing, but also extremely powerful. What gives the eating disorder this power? What makes eating disorders so important to those who suffer from them. What meaning and value do young people give to their disorders? These are questions we need to answer if we are to banish this Wicked Witch and help our children to become healthy again.

THE INTENSITY OF THE EATING DISORDER

In an article written in 1998, Kelly Vitousek discusses how difficult it is for an outside observer to understand the control an eating disorder can have on someone. She asks a young father to imagine being faced with the following situation:

"I am a psychologist who specializes in the detection and prevention of unhealthy relationships between parents and children," she began. "After careful assessment of your family, I am convinced that it was a terrible mistake for you to have your (baby) daughter. You may feel quite attached to her at the moment, but in the long run it simply won't work out. Whatever pleasure you may think you are getting out of the relationship, a detached and objective observer can see that you are losing a great deal, too. You are tired and run down, you lack sufficient energy for many of the activities you used to find rewarding, you spend less time with you friends, and sometimes your work has suffered. You have become so preoccupied with this child that you are unable to make a realistic assessment of how she has actually affected your life.

"Therefore, I have decided to take your daughter away. I can appreciate that you feel angry with me just now, and may not believe it is my right to interfere — but eventually you will come to understand that I have acted in your own best interest. With your child gone you will be able to return to the life you had before you became a parent."

This father likely already understands the difficulties that come with having a new baby. These sacrifices, however, will pale in comparison to the love he has for his daughter and his drive to protect that child at all costs. Indeed, if someone were to try and take his baby daughter away, the father might go to extreme lengths to shelter her.

The eating disorder may be just as precious to your child. Young people may have great difficulty understanding why everyone is asking them to give up something they feel is so vitally important and worth protecting.

The Meaning of the Eating Disorder

An eating disorder may have begun with a simple diet in an attempt to lose weight to meet a social ideal. Our society values weight loss, where having a low weight for your height is a value to be supported and a way to feel accepted by others. Losing weight presents a number of rewards.

Eating Disorder Pride

For teenagers with perfectionistic tendencies, the diet becomes a major focus. When they lose weight, they often receive praise for their efforts. "I have never been able to do what you seem to have done," a parent, family member, or friend may remark. Weight loss and food restriction soon become a ready source of pride, value, and self-esteem. (This is not true for all people. Many young people truly wish that no one would notice them. Even if it is true, your child may not be fully aware of this.)

In addition, because of the value our society places on losing weight, they may feel morally righteous or pure. They may go on to believe that others are secretly jealous of them, which, they reason, may be why everyone is now recommending they gain weight for their health. The eating disorder may then provide them with a feeling of being unique. Weight and shape become an essential way of assessing their worth as a person. Over time, this feeling of being special can provide a new source of identity. This might be something that the person had never felt before, and it leaves them with a strong sense of purpose.

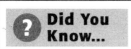
Did You Know...

• Most teenagers will attempt to diet; for someone who develops an eating disorder, however, this diet ends up taking on new meaning.

• This new meaning initiates the strong attachment between the person and the eating disorder.

Eating Disorder Power

Other unexpected advantages may arise that serve as strong reasons to hold onto the eating disorder. Children and adolescents with eating disorders may discover the power they have within their family. They may feel that they are strong within themselves and have control over something for the first time in their lives. If they enjoy this feeling of power, they may feel that they are only able to express it through the eating disorder, though not in other areas of their life, such as at school or with their friends. This makes the eating disorder more profound.

WORKSHEET

WHAT CAN THE EATING DISORDER MEAN TO YOUR CHILD?

The following list offers a glimpse at the possible meanings we have heard young people give to their eating disorders. Working with your child, you might try checking off any of these meanings that your child has given to the eating disorder. Not every child gives all of these meanings to the eating disorder, so only one or more (or perhaps none) may apply to your child. Younger children may have difficulty recognizing or vocalizing a meaning.

☐ I am now unique and special.

☐ I feel virtuous and pure.

☐ Not eating allows me to feel in complete control of my life.

☐ Not eating makes me feel happy — right away!

☐ This makes me feel that I can do what no one else can.

☐ Eating means I am a failure.

☐ Eating means that I am weak.

☐ I need to punish myself by not eating.

☐ I don't deserve to eat. If I eat, I don't deserve to go to a movie.

☐ Not eating allows me to be the center of attention.

☐ Not eating allows all my other worries to go away. This is all I have to focus on.

☐ When I don't eat, I divert attention away from other events, e.g., arguments at home. (For some children, not eating may be how they choose to cope with arguments.)

☐ When I don't eat, I feel empty. This feels comfortable.

☐ Not eating allows me to lose my period. I don't want my period.

☐ I don't want to grow up.

☐ The eating disorder is who I am.

Eating Disorder Hurt

At the same time, children and adolescents with eating disorders may feel upset at how hurtful they are becoming. This worry makes them feel worse about themselves. When they feel badly about themselves, they may turn to the eating disorder as the way of coping they know best. The cycle then continues.

Eating Disorder Protection

Other advantages may also seem to arise. They may find that their emotions are numbed and that their other worries become less significant. The eating disorder becomes all that they have to focus on. Over time, the disorder becomes something that is familiar and therefore comforting. Not eating becomes equated with feeling good about oneself, being in control, being happy. The eating disorder may become a way of organizing life, especially for those who crave simplicity and predictability. It can also protect young people from the fear of growing up and maturing.

Vicious Circles

As further weight loss is achieved, or the binge and purge cycle progresses, the child or adolescent enters a world where starvation itself affects the thought processes. Thoughts start to become obsessive; it is difficult for the person to focus on anything other than the eating disorder. These thoughts then allow the behavior and illness to become stronger.

Obsession

With obsessive thinking, people become more anxious, worrying about whether they are eating too much or are getting fat, thinking more and more about their obsessions. Frequently, the only way that they feel they can reduce the anxiety associated with their obsession is by further restricting food.

Self-Worth

Perfectionism creates its own trappings. When the attempt is to be 'flawless', each time a person inevitably 'fails', it brings out feelings of low self-worth. This, too, will often lead to further convictions and increased restriction of food.

Control

The acts of binging and purging have their own unique reinforcers. A binge is accompanied by a feeling of loss of control, and young people with eating disorders may use further restriction as an attempt to regain control and feel good

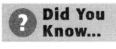

Did You Know...

• During times of increased stress, young people may turn to the eating disorder because it has appeared to help them reduce their anxiety in the past.

• These thoughts are very powerful.

about themselves. As restriction will inevitably lead to another binge, they, too, get caught in an endless cycle. They may also start to feel they are not good enough to perfect 'not eating', and therefore attempt to restrict their eating more vigorously. Purging often results from the powerful guilt feelings that follow a binge. It may also have the effect of numbing emotions, or "vomiting everything that is evil inside." Binging itself may numb emotions, as well as satisfy intense cravings.

Effects of Starvation

Much of the power of an eating disorder comes from the effects of starvation on the mind and body. There is an incredible resemblance between victims of starvation (who do not have the wish to be thin) and individuals with an eating disorders.

One of the best studies demonstrating the effects of starvation on the mind was conducted by Ancel Keys and his colleagues at the University of Minnesota during World War II. They took 36 young men, who had volunteered for the study as an alternative to military service, and put them on a severe diet. For 3 months, their behavior, personality, and eating patterns were studied in detail while they ate a normal diet. In the following 6 months, the men were given half of their former food intake. They lost an average of 25% of their body weight. This was followed by a 3-month rehabilitation phase of gradually re-feeding the men.

While the individual responses to this state of semi-starvation varied, most of the men experienced significant physical, psychological, and social changes. They all had been deemed mentally healthy at the outset of the study and were considered to have superior "psycholobiological stamina." In most cases, these changes lasted throughout rehabilitation and, in some cases, longer.

The study also demonstrated that binging is the body's natural response to restriction. As we now know, up to 30% of people with anorexia nervosa will go on to develop binge and purge symptoms or bulimia nervosa.

EFFECTS OF SEMI-STARVATION: KEYS STUDY

Food Preoccupation
- Food becomes the principal topic of conversation, reading, and dreams
- Change of career plans (e.g., to become chefs)
- Hoarding of food and non-food related items

Eating Habits Changes
(persisted during re-feeding)
- Started to eat in silence, preoccupied with eating process
- Prolonged time ingesting food
- Great increase in use of salt and spices
- Unusual mixing and combinations of food
- Excessive gum chewing
- Excessive ingestion of coffee and tea

Emotional Changes
(persisted during re-feeding and became worse for some)
- Depression
- Irritability
- Frequent outbursts of anger
- Extreme mood swings
- High levels of anxiety (including nail biting)
- Almost 20% experienced extreme emotional deterioration (some were hospitalized)

Social Changes
- Men became withdrawn
- Decreased desire to socialize
- Less humor
- Diminished sexual interests

Cognitive Changes
(ability to think and reason)
- Impaired concentration
- Less alert
- Lack of comprehension
- Failing judgment

Bulimia
(for some men, bulimia persisted for many months after free access to food)
- Episodes of binging and vomiting, when given more free access to food
- Binging felt "out of control"

WORKSHEET

PSYCHOLOGICAL COMPLICATIONS OF EATING DISORDERS

Eating disorders can cause a variety of psychological changes. Use this worksheet to check off any changes in mood and behavior you have witnessed with your child.

☐ Poor concentration   ☐ Mood fluctuations

☐ Poor problem solving   ☐ Difficulty sleeping

☐ Poor planning   ☐ Crying spells

☐ Irritability   ☐ Loss of interest in regular activities

☐ Anxiety   ☐ Withdrawal from family and friends

☐ Sadness   ☐ Thoughts of self-harm

Behavior and Mood Changes

Children and adolescents with eating disorders show similar physical, psychological, and social changes from the effects of semi-starvation as the men in the Keys study. Many of the abnormal behaviors common in adolescents with eating disorders are a result of starvation, not personality or 'teenage' behavior. These emotional and thinking changes can radically change personality and the way a person functions in the world.

The stubbornness or aggressiveness these children and adolescents demonstrate may be highly affected by their state of starvation. Indeed, underneath a harsh exterior, adolescents suffering with eating disorders are usually extremely scared. This behavior, as one author explains, is the "response of someone who is frightened, hurt, and extraordinarily unhappy."

In addition, the development of depression can make it harder to recover from the illness. Individuals can start to live in their own world, forgetting all the other pleasures that they once enjoyed. The young person may feel pessimistic that there is no other way of living.

The effects on one's ability to think and reason are also striking. At worst, young people can get locked into irrational thinking and poor judgment. They may think in an "all or nothing" way, such as: "If I eat one chip, I might as well give up and have a whole binge" or "Unless I'm thinner than everyone else, I'm fat and therefore worthless." Their ability to understand what they are doing may be truly impaired.

The Voice

Many adolescents who suffer with an eating disorder will identify with 'the voice' of the disorder. The eating disorder takes on its own identity and seems to talk directly to the person. "If you eat that, you're weak," it may say. "If you do what I say, you'll become successful." This voice can be so powerful that it becomes the only thing your child hears. It drowns out all other voices, all rational thought. It has a powerful way of saying, "Your feelings don't matter...all that matters is to be in control."

The eating disorder becomes an outside force that has a powerful way of becoming your child's closest ally. It has a way of making young people feel like it is the only thing that they can trust. This may start with advantages the child feels from dieting and be strengthened by the effects of starvation.

Adolescents who have lived with an eating disorder can sometimes recognize that the eating disorder is both "tricky" and "slippery." Some call it "the devil" or other negative names, even though part of them continues to feel it is their best friend. When asked how it becomes so powerful, they respond by explaining, "It takes advantage of girls and boys who like to do the best or be the best" or "It takes over their

WHAT THE EATING DISORDER 'VOICE' MIGHT SAY

- "Don't eat."

- "You're weak if you eat."

- "You're dumb if you eat."

- "You are fat and do not deserve to eat."

- "The only hope for you is to stay disciplined and become thin."

- "If only you lose 10 more pounds."

- "Be strong, don't give in."

- "It doesn't matter what anyone else tells you, those rules don't apply to you. I won't let you get sick."

- "Those people don't really care about you."

- "You're actually getting stronger, not weaker."

CASE STUDY Martha

Martha spent time looking in the mirror every time she went to the bathroom. She couldn't help it — her bathroom had floor-to-ceiling mirrors. Every time she looked in the mirror she heard the voice saying, "fat, fat, fat."

The voice in her head kept telling her that she was a failure unless she lost weight. When she did lose weight, she felt successful — at least for a few moments. Then the voice said, "Not enough, you need to lose more weight…what happens if one day you eat too much and gain weight? If you lose more now, you'll have a buffer."

So, one night after dinner she went to the bathroom and looked in the mirror…all she could see was a fat belly. Even though she knew she was hurting herself and her parents, she had to throw up…she had to get rid of the food. She had to do something about all this fat!

The voice in her head kept reminding her, "Nothing was worse than being fat!" In desperation, she turned on the tap and bent over the toilet.

continued on page 103

mind completely." One young woman stated, "It takes away things that I used to know were true."

Similar to the Wicked Witch in Snow White, the eating disorder can successfully hide its 'evil' intentions. It can be hard for a person to recognize that this 'wonderful' eating disorder is directly causing them to lose their friends, to become depressed, and to harm themselves physically.

Acting Against the Voice

Even if your child does not identify with a voice per se, thinking of the eating disorder as an outside force can be very helpful in understanding its power. For example, it allows a parent to understand mood changes during meals as a result of the eating disorder taking over, not as a deliberate act of defiance. This approach can then make it easier to talk with your child directly and provide support. It can make it easier for everyone on your health-care team (and eventually your child) to be on the same side, working against the eating disorder. For your child, it can start to reverse the process of self-blame: "It's the eating disorder's fault!" For others, it helps them to question our culture in general and not blame the child directly. Focusing anger at Snow White is unlikely to make the Witch leave. Supporting Snow White, however, can help her guide the Wicked Witch out the door.

Recovery Hurdles

"The willpower to stop eating," one young person with an eating order remarked, "was the easy part compared to the willpower needed to get better." Once young people with an eating disorder choose to act against the eating disorder, it truly is not a matter of just regaining their weight or a vowing to never binge or purge again. In addition to giving up the 'benefits' of an eating disorder and allowing time for the effects of starvation to pass, there are other hurdles that make the recovery process difficult to face.

Phobic Foods

By the time the eating disorder has set in, simply eating, especially certain 'phobic' foods, has become your child's worst nightmare. Recovery is usually a matter of very gradually facing fears and getting used to regular eating patterns and these phobic foods. This takes a leap of faith no less trying than overcoming phobias to spiders, snakes, and heights.

Eating Pain

The process can also be physically uncomfortable because the person's body is not accustomed to the regular intake of food. Your child may experience swelling and bloating as a result of re-feeding. This can reassert the fear of eating. The only treatment for this stomach upset is to keep eating and gradually increase the amount of food. This will give the stomach a chance to get used to working normally again.

Eating Disorder Addiction

An eating disorder has its own addictive quality as well. People frequently talk about a 'high' from fasting, in that it feels like a habit or a drug. Similar to a person recovering from alcoholism, needing to give up drinking forever, a person wanting to recover from an eating disorder will need to get rid of many of their triggers, such as scales, friends who diet, and diet foods. This can be very difficult when our culture reinforces so many of these triggers.

Fear of Change

One last hurdle for the adolescent with an eating disorder is a tremendous fear of change. An eating disorder may have become the only thing that they know; it may have created a complete sense of who they are. It may be an important mechanism to manage their emotions, a way of making them feel good about themselves and in control. Change can be uncomfortable and very, very difficult. New and healthier ways of feeling good and handling emotions will need to be developed.

CASE STUDY Martha

After a long discussion with the family therapist, Martha's parents decided that she should start individual therapy. This might help her sort out her own issues. Not long after that decision was made, Martha got caught shoplifting. Her parents were humiliated when they picked her up from the mall. The charges were dropped because she had a mental illness. Martha's parents were surprised to discover that kids with bulimia nervosa also had problems called impulse control. These impulse control problems explained the drinking and shoplifting. They now understood that the eating disorder was part of Martha's struggle as a person.

They hoped that through her work with the individual therapist, she would learn how to manage her feelings, impulses, and desires. Martha's mother blamed herself for Martha's eating disorder and this impulse control problem. She acknowledged that she spoiled Martha, who was the youngest child in their family and the only girl. The doctors explained that some of this was likely due to Martha's character, and with therapy, she could learn how to change her thinking and behavior.

continued on page 147

How Could This Have Happened to Our Family?

A Mother's Story

IT ALL STARTED INNOCENTLY ENOUGH. WHEN OUR 15-YEAR-OLD daughter announced one day that she wanted to pursue healthier eating habits, we were thrilled. She had arrived at adolescence with a few extra pounds gained primarily through an overactive sweet tooth, and we all believed it was never too early to develop good lifetime habits. First, she cut out sweets and snack foods, then beef, then meat of any kind, soon followed by all carbohydrates. She seemed to be living primarily on water and fruit salad. She also indicated that she had started exercising, which translated, unbeknown to us, into 3-hour daily walks and at least 400 sit-ups a day. She was mesmerized by every mirror she passed, pulling in her stomach and checking her profile at every opportunity.

The weight started to come off pretty quickly, but we only became alarmed after a 5-day trip to New York City, where she walked all day, ate virtually nothing, and lost 8 pounds. Fortunately, at that time we had an excellent contact at the children's hospital in our city, who referred us to a psychologist specializing in the treatment of adolescents with eating-related problems. Although I had read several books about young girls and the many challenges they faced as their bodies began to change, we were unprepared to call it an actual eating disorder. She developed an excellent relationship with this therapist as together they explored issues of body image, distorted media depictions of young women, and unrealistic societal expectations, but the weight continued to drop.

She was mesmerized by every mirror she passed, pulling in her stomach and checking her profile at every opportunity.

A few months into treatment, the therapist recommended medical intervention. Our pediatrician, alarmed at the sight of our daughter after an absence of several months, immediately took steps to refer her to the Eating Disorder Program at the children's hospital. Our previous experiences with the hospital had us convinced that this was the best program in the city, but we knew that being seen would be very difficult because of a lengthy waiting list.

While we waited, our doctor insisted on a weekly electrocardiogram (EKG). The EKG is a graphic tracing of the electrical activity of the heart muscle and this was used to monitor her heart function. One evening, after one of these routine tests, he called to direct us immediately to the emergency room of the hospital. Apparently, her heart rate was so irregular and so slow that she was in imminent danger of collapse. We went as instructed, fully believing we would be coming home soon. Our dismay was therefore so much greater when we were told that she was being admitted that night to the Eating Disorder Program's inpatient ward.

As I approached the ward that shared space with the psychiatric short-term care facility, I was overcome with the feeling that I had walked through the looking glass. I had no real understanding of what had happened and why we were still there. My husband went home in a daze of disbelief, while I was allowed to spend that first night with my daughter. Her heart monitor, set to sound the alarm every time her heart rate fell below 40 beat per minute, went off periodically through the night. As I lay listening to it, I could only wonder how my child, my baby, could have come to this, lying in a hospital bed hooked up to wires that would tell us if her heart was about to stop beating.

Apparently, her heart rate was so irregular and so slow that she was in imminent danger of collapse.

Although she was seen in those first hours and days by a medical army that included doctors, students, psychiatrists, psychologists, nurses, social workers, youth workers, and teachers, we had absolutely no idea what the treatment plan would be, nor how long she would be hospitalized. All we were really told in the beginning was that she would be restricted to her bed until her heart stabilized and would remain on the ward until she reached 85% of her ideal body weight. Who knew then what that weight was even supposed to be?

Little did I realize at that time that three years and four hospitalizations later, I would know more than I ever cared to about eating disorders, their causes, and courses of treatment.

What do we tell our friends and family...

After initially balking at the idea of staying in hospital and repeated bouts of tears, our daughter finally accepted the idea that she was not going home right away. Her first concern was school. She had always been an excellent, hard-driving student and, assuming she would only be in hospital a few days, did not want to fall behind. She asked me to collect work, but not to divulge the true nature of her illness. She had an underlying chronic medical condition, and insisted we tell people that complications from that illness were causing her absence from school. She swore us to absolute secrecy on the truth. We, however, felt that we needed the support of friends and family to get through the ordeal that I sensed was awaiting us and chose to tell those closest to us. In retrospect, this two-pronged approach failed miserably. After a while, I could no longer remember which lie I had told when and to whom. My husband chose to tell anyone who would listen, hoping to uncover a similar story that had ended well. I wanted to tell those whom I felt would support me. We both had to keep these confidences a secret from our daughter.

Everyone who knew the truth had 'valuable' advice to give: "Of course, she doesn't eat. Look at you; you have been dieting your whole life." "If you all had modeled better eating habits, this would not have happened." "Just tell her to eat. She's a smart girl; she'll listen." "Don't tell anyone the truth. People will think she is mentally ill and she will never get a job, a boyfriend, a husband."

Everyone who knew the truth had 'valuable' advice to give: "Of course, she doesn't eat. Look at you; you have been dieting your whole life."

For a mother already feeling immense guilt over the plight of her child, nothing could have been worse. No one understood at the time that this was an illness like many others, and it became too exhausting to try to explain. I slowly began to distance myself from my friends. Not wanting to hear their advice, however well-intended, it was easier to return calls briefly from the car on my way home and pretend that everything was fine.

As for the three of us, the immediate family, we each started spinning in our own orbit, trying in our own unique way to cope. Our son, away at university, distanced himself from the problem by rarely calling or visiting, in an attempt to minimize his own pain. My husband immersed himself in work and only surfaced to visit his daughter every day. Satisfied with the information he was receiving from the medical team, he was confident she was in the best possible hands and needed little more. Ever doubtful that I had done enough, I went on a frantic search of the Internet, looking for alternative treatment options, case histories, and success stories, which, in retrospect, I realize was an attempt to mitigate my own guilt and feelings of helplessness. Unfortunately, it seems that few people bother to share happy news on the Net. I only found stories of disappointment and failure, serving only to deepen those negative emotions.

How to be a better anorexic...

Convinced she was only going to be on the ward a few days, our daughter decided that cooperation was her best option. She quickly learned the routines of the ward and made friends with some of the girls who were there for a third and fourth time. After she was released from bed rest, I usually found her in the ward lounge. I walked in one day to find them all madly knitting, like Madame Defarge on speed. What they were making they could not say, but I was told it was good therapy. They all had their legs crossed at the knee, with one leg frantically bobbing up and down. I later learned that this was another attempt to burn off any calories they had consumed.

Communal meals resulted in their learning from one another how to hide food from the watchful eyes of nurses. We had been told that most of the young people who succumb to eating disorders are very bright. Watching them put their energies toward finding creative and ingenious ways to avoid the treatments that had been prescribed, I could not help feeling that they were all better suited to a life of espionage. In truth, they all seemed to feel that they were perfectly healthy, certainly not suffering from an eating disorder, and that their hospitalization was a conspiracy between their parents and staff to make them fat.

In truth, they all seemed to feel that they were perfectly healthy, certainly not suffering from an eating disorder, and that their hospitalization was a conspiracy between their parents and staff to make them fat.

Although our daughter wanted desperately to resume her normal life, every morning's weigh-in was traumatic. Every ounce of weight gained took her closer to her objective of leaving the hospital but farther from her goal of the perfect body. Even on the ward she compared herself to the others; seemingly, her aspiration was to be the slimmest one there and thereby the 'best' anorexic.

What have you done with my daughter...

As she descended further and further into her illness, our daughter became a virtual stranger. She and I had always taken pride in our closeness and considered ourselves not just mother and daughter but best friends. Although she seemed to need me while in hospital, we would have the fiercest battles of our relationship.

While she was on the ward, the hospital was responsible for her caloric intake. When she was finally given evening passes, we would go to a movie and then she was allowed to have evening snack with me. This became a negotiation. She knew what the required foods were and tried as much as possible to bargain that amount down.

The long-awaited weekend pass was a true test of our relationship. While anxious to come home, she was depressed from the start because she knew the weekend would end and she would have to go back on Sunday. Every meal was a battle. We had left the ward armed with a weekend meal plan that went out the window at the first meal. Not wanting to spend the short period fighting, I would struggle to hold my tongue, all the while knowing that her weight was dropping. I was more than a little relieved to deliver her back to the ward on Sunday night, to the waiting arms of nurses who were not emotionally involved. We left each other feeling guilty, I for wanting to hand off the responsibility to someone else, she for having failed at a simple weekend outing.

When she was home, we watched her like hawks. We negotiated and argued over every mouthful.

We repeated this dance on almost every weekend pass. She felt that she was eating plenty; we knew it was not enough. By Monday morning, she had usually lost weight. This just made her angrier because it was prolonging the hospitalization. Yet her anger was mixed with relief at not having become 'fat' over the weekend. We could not understand her behavior, which appeared to us completely counter-intuitive. We would ask: "If you want to come home, why don't you just eat?" She would respond: "I can come home and handle this myself. There is nothing wrong with me."

When she was home, we watched her like hawks. We negotiated and argued over every mouthful. I tried begging and pleading; her father ended up shouting in sheer frustration. Everyone walked on eggshells. We had been told that the path to recovery was in her hands. She would start down that road only when she was ready. If only we could muster the patience to wait.

Seeking more help...

The hospital provided us with considerable support. We participated in group counseling sessions, which, while informative, scared me to death. At these meetings, I met parents whose children, usually daughters, were in hospital for the sixth and seventh time. I tried to listen only to the positive stories, but there were so few of them. I would go home at night worrying that she would never go to university, never hold down a job, never find a mate or be able to have children, that she would be in and out of hospital her entire life, and that all the hopes and dreams I had for her, developed over 9 months in the womb and her first 15 years of life, would come to naught, that they would vanish forever into the maw of this insidious illness. I knew this line of thinking was not productive, but it was impossible to still those voices in the middle of the night.

Under the guidance of two very caring, compassionate, and competent therapists, we learned a great deal about our family dynamics.

Inevitably, we befriended other parents during our daily visits to the ward. As we exchanged confidences and related our experiences, it became clear that, while the girls shared many similarities, no two stories were exactly alike. Some ended in tragedy; others promised a happier outcome. These strangers were the only people who really understood when we spoke in the jargon of the eating disorder ward. We had all learned a secret language, to which our real-life friends were not privy. We seemed to exist in a parallel universe.

When our daughter was ready, we participated in family therapy. Under the guidance of two very caring, compassionate, and competent therapists, we learned a great deal about our family dynamics. We had always known that we were a closely-knit unit, likely overprotective of one another (a possible by-product of our Eastern European, post-Holocaust heritage). We learned that we were all resistant to change, that she, while wanting to grow up, was somehow afraid of the separation from family that adolescence would entail, and that we, in turn, were having difficulty adapting to her growing up. It was made clear to us that we had not caused our daughter's eating disorder, and that she would have to find her own way out. Our role was to support her and adapt to the changing family dynamic that would accompany her recovery.

In addition, the program provided our daughter with individual counseling, both on an inpatient and outpatient basis.

This was probably the most helpful element of her treatment. She established an immediate rapport with her therapist, and together, over many months and through multiple hospitalizations, they explored issues of friendship, family, school, societal expectations, sexuality, self-esteem, and all the other subjects that can plague the life of an adolescent. Our daughter came to rely heavily on these sessions as she tried to fight her way out of her illness.

It was made clear to us that we had not caused our daughter's eating disorder, and that she would have to find her own way out.

In contrast, the least helpful component of the treatment plan was the psychiatric intervention. Two psychiatrists were involved during the process, neither of whom was able to establish much of a relationship with our daughter. Perhaps this was not their job or perhaps she was just resistant to their methods. Their principal role was to prescribe and monitor medication, which ultimately became necessary and useful — another implement in the toolbox for recovery.

She did not like the group therapy much better. She had difficulty sharing personal thoughts with virtual strangers, and, although the girls came to rely heavily on one another, they never became actual confidantes. This illness had drawn them together, but life had treated them all very differently.

The final straw...

By the time of her fourth hospitalization, the program was changed to include longer stays, higher target discharge weights, and a graduated allowance of ward privileges. This was an improvement over the previous system, in that it gave patients a much greater degree of control over their recovery. The more they cooperated, the faster they gained weight and the more freedom they were given. Unfortunately, by this time, our daughter was in no mood to cooperate.

Before this fourth hospitalization, she had been given several warnings that if her weight continued to drop during her weekly outpatient visits to the clinic, her doctors would have no choice but to keep her there. Since she had always been so cooperative, so sweet, and so convincing in her promises to do better, always accompanied by huge crocodile tears, she repeatedly managed to persuade all of us — parents, medical staff, therapists — that this time, she would gain the weight on her own. Everyone wanted to give her the benefit of the doubt. However, after the fourth consecutive weekly loss, we all insisted that she stay.

She rebelled for the first time, so vehemently and so violently that she had to be threatened with security guards and restraints. I could not recognize this young woman who was screaming that she hated me and would never forgive me, and who was being so belligerent with a doctor she otherwise adored. Although restraints and the guard proved unnecessary, the experience left us all shaken and questioning the wisdom of our decision.

She rebelled for the first time, so vehemently and so violently that she had to be threatened with security guards and restraints.

Once she finally accepted confinement to the ward again, she took on a leadership role among the other patients. Since this was her fourth stay, some of the others looked to her for guidance. Her 12-year-old roommate called her a role model and another patient who had been in different hospitals before landing at this children's hospital found her to be one of the few people in whom he could confide. Trying to help others seemed to advance her own healing, although this was fraught with its own ups and downs. Her weight at this time was likely the highest of all on the ward and this caused her considerable anxiety, far more than the unstable heart that had resulted in this hospitalization.

At this point, she was just starting her final year of high school. Her doctors, understanding the importance she attached to school, allowed her to go to school once she reached her 85% target and come back to the hospital for meals and to sleep. This strategy worked for a while until one day, in a fit of anger over something one of her doctors had said, she took an extra long walk (or several) and managed to lose two pounds in two days. The medical staff issued their ultimatum: stop going to school, stay in hospital, and concentrate on getting well or go home for good. To our surprise, she struggled with this decision for several hours. We knew how much she hated the inflexibility of the new system and how badly she wanted to go home. Yet clearly she was afraid of taking that irrevocable step. She finally decided that going home was her best option, but things were very slow to improve. For every two steps she took forward, she took half as many backwards. We were all desperate. She was approaching her 18th birthday and would have to move to the adult system, which frightened all of us.

During this last stay in hospital I had asked her doctor if she thought our daughter would ever get well. I found her answer less than reassuring: "Yes, eventually, but I can't tell you when. It could take a very long time and she will only get better when she wants to." Never one to be able to live with uncertainty, I started a desperate search for another answer. I sought out alternative facilities with residential programs (finding nothing that appealed to me) and haunted the bookstores for writers I could relate to. On one of these visits I found a book by a New York City therapist who had devoted his career to the treatment of eating disorders. The case histories in the book related perfectly to our own experiences and reflected much of the treatment plan we had experienced. I found him on the Internet and requested an appointment.

> *For every two steps she took forward, she took half as many backwards.*

By this time, after two-and-a-half years of living with this affliction, I would have gone anywhere in the world and would have spent any amount of money for a solution. I was grateful that we only had to go to New York!

The light at the end of the tunnel...
We waited 6 weeks for the appointment. During that period, we began to notice small changes. For a very long time, our daughter had avoided many of her school friends and had consistently refused any invitations to sleepovers. Suddenly one weekend, she asked to have a friend stay overnight at our home. Hearing noises at 3:00 a.m., I went down to the kitchen to find them both eating cookies by the handful. I was in shock. She had not voluntarily had a cookie in almost 3 years, much less a cream-filled one!

By the time we went to New York, she was eating sweets again, although it was instead of regular food. Her session with the therapist was a big success and served to reinforce everything that had been done to that point. Coming on the heels of a steadily improving eating pattern, we went home feeling quite optimistic. In the days and weeks following the visit, all the elements of the multipronged approach to her treatment seemed to come together.

As she continued to eat, the daughter we had always known started to re-emerge. Of course, being a child of extremes, she started eating more sweets and less 'real' food. During her weekly visits to the clinic, she was learning *how* to eat again. As a vegetarian, getting sufficient protein was a challenge, but at this point, we didn't really care; any food consumed was most welcome.

She offered no explanation for the change. She claimed something had just snapped and she was tired of the effort required to be anorexic. By the time she graduated from the program on her 18th birthday, she was at 100% of her target weight, looking forward to a family cruise (despite the mountains of food that cruising offers) and to starting university out of town in the fall.

As she continued to eat, the daughter we had always known started to re-emerge. Of course, being a child of extremes, she started eating more sweets and less 'real' food.

Food will always be a challenge, as it is for so many people. She still worries about her weight, still resorts to extremes of eating and exercising when she is not feeling in perfect control of her life, and will still sometimes compare herself unfavorably to friends and even strangers. Although the struggle with body image is not over, we are delighted that her tenacity and force of will helped put her on the road to recovery well ahead of schedule. We can only hope that she now has the tools to confront those challenges without doing herself further physical harm.

Now what do I do...

While my daughter was ill, I knew exactly what my role was. I needed to look after and support her, attend to my household, and continue to run my business. Once she was recovering and off to university, I was bereft. With my house empty, I couldn't find my place. Clearly, I needed to re-define my own role.

One year and many hours of individual therapy later, I periodically enjoy the solitude of my home, have taken the opportunity to travel, and am embarking on a new career. The past 3 years have forced a change in all of us, and now that we have emerged on the other side of our ordeal, we are a stronger family for the effort. So many times, when we were tempted to give up, we encountered people — the medical staff, other parents — who pushed us to keep on fighting. We are grateful for their encouragement and learned a valuable lesson: the light at the end of the tunnel, though dim at times, is never out.

DOs AND DON'Ts FOR PARENTS

Here is some hard-earned advice that may help you as a parent and your child cope with the eating disorder.

Do

- Do seek medical advice as soon as you notice an abnormal change in eating or exercise habits or a dramatic loss of weight in a short period of time.

- Do seek a second opinion if your health-care professional does not take this seriously.

- Do praise your child for non-eating-related accomplishments.

- Do take what you read on the Internet with a grain of salt; very few people post good news.

- Do keep up the fight; recovery is a long process.

- Do have trust in your medical team. They have the resources and experience to see you through this crisis.

Don't

- Don't nag your child to eat; this will only make him or her angry. Let the health-care professionals be the 'bad guys'.

- Don't be offended by your child's outbursts of anger – even if they are directed at you. They are using you as an outlet for anger that is often directed at them.

- Don't allow yourself to be drawn into arguments that neither of you can win; this only leads to more anger and frustration.

- Don't comment on your child's appearance; this will only be received as criticism.

- Don't compare your child to anyone else; no two cases are exactly alike.

- Don't talk endlessly with your adolescent about the eating disorder. Try to find activities that you can enjoy together and that do not involve food.

- Don't be discouraged...most young people with eating disorders recover!

PART 2

Treating Eating Disorders

...harting the Road to Recovery

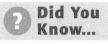
Now that we have an understanding of what eating disorders are, the factors that lead to their development, as well as the serious medical and psychological consequences that may develop because of progressive weight loss and disordered eating, we can begin to chart a course for treatment and recovery. A medical assessment of your child and your family will be the first clinical step in this process, followed by a choice of treatment strategies and facilities, but before any program can succeed, there is a need to create a mind-set to support your child through the natural course of recovery from the eating. The road to recovery has several challenging stages or phases that can best be navigated if we have the right mind-set.

Like a courageous mountain climber at base camp, you may now clearly see the challenge that lies before you. You know that you and your child have to climb and conquer that mountain (because it's there!). You've studied the maps found in your reading and research. Now, you are ready to explore different routes up the mountain, different approaches to the summit. But your child may not yet be ready to follow. You will likely begin to feel like you're stumbling rather than climbing, alone. Instead of having your child as an able member of your climb team, you may frequently feel as though you are dragging your daughter or son up the steepest slopes, only to watch them willingly tumble back down to where you first began your ascent.

You knew that climbing this mountain wouldn't be a 'walk in the park', but you also know this mountain has been successfully scaled by many that have come before you. What's going on here? What's going wrong?

Two Mind-sets

There are two main obstacles that threaten your success. The first is the nature of the mountain — the eating disorder itself. The climbing conditions seem to change so unpredictably from day to day. A certain path that shows promise today ends up at an impasse tomorrow. You will need lots of perseverance and patience.

The second obstacle is the attitude of your fellow climber. Your child with the eating disorder thinks that the whole expedition is unnecessary and misguided. Your son or daughter wants to drop the whole thing. They never really agreed to do this with you in the first place, did they? You will need even more perseverance and patience.

Let's look at ways to overcome these obstacles and resolve the difference between your mind-set and your child's mind-set.

Traditional Medical Mind-set

First, we need to let go of the mindset we traditionally bring to bear upon anyone who is medically ill. You may now believe that your child is suffering from various symptoms of a serious disorder. Your child has become or is becoming physically and psychologically unwell. You may assume that your child's experience of the symptoms of this illness must be distressing (as you can see that yourself). Your child must want to become well again. Seeking treatment in order to alleviate the symptoms of this illness and restore the previous state of good health is in order.

These assumptions are all accurate when faced with someone complaining of a medical condition like asthma or an acute physical symptom like diarrhea. For eating disorders, especially in the early phases, these assumptions simply do not apply to what your child believes. In almost any other medical or psychiatric disorder, an adolescent would be distressed by the symptoms and would want to have the pain taken away by immediate professional treatment. For example, adolescents who are experiencing serious social anxiety, who are fearful of all unfamiliar social situations, who avoid being the focus of attention at all costs, and who prefer to isolate themselves in their bedroom after school, readily admit to their emotional distress and welcome assistance that promises to help them let go of their fears, overcome debilitating anxieties, and discover a far happier way of living their lives. These adolescents also make no effort to disguise their symptoms.

The Eating Disorder Mind-set

Adolescents with eating disorders often make a great effort to conceal and deny the nature and severity of their symptoms. Later on, even once their eating disorder behaviors and attitudes have been exposed to your family, they may continue to avoid, resist, and reject the efforts from anyone who dares to try to help them find treatments to overcome their illness and restore them their previous state of health. These young people defy our expectations about illness by showing no desire to get better.

Following the traditional medical path from diagnosis through treatment to recovery becomes an impasse. To force your traditional assumptions about illness on your son or daughter when they wholly reject the idea that they are sick and then to demand that they just get better and start eating will not be received as supportive. It may even be seen as punitive and uncaring.

If this rings true for the situation with your child, then you're probably asking: "What is it about eating disorders that tend to defy our usual assumptions about being sick and about getting better?" To help answer this, consider another way of understanding what your child may be going through.

Shifting Point of View

Seeing the world from your child's point of view should help you to understand why your daughter or son has been acting so unlike their 'real' self, so full of unpredictable behaviors, moods, and attitudes that are confusing to everyone and that end up hurting them and your whole family.

In your son's or your daughter's mind-set, they are behaving in a way that is both sensible and adaptive to their present needs. At least in the beginning months, their reasons for pursuing the eating disorder must be providing something very rewarding. You may already be thinking: "How could having the disordered behaviors and beliefs of an eating disorder, including the risks of developing dangerous medical consequences, be in any way sensible and adaptive, not to mention rewarding, for my child?"

Sociocultural Factors

Recall for a moment the sociocultural factors we have seen influencing the development of eating disorders. First, adolescents live in the midst of a marketing-heavy, pop culture that is particularly intent on pairing up everything that is cool, desirable, and critical for adolescent success with an endless stream of teen idols (e.g., models, musicians, actors) who are chosen just as much for their attractive, marketable image as for their talent.

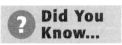

Did You Know...

● As bizarre as it sounds, the initial pathway toward an eating disorder does come with a number of physical, psychological, and social rewards.

● These rewards are highly prized by any adolescent.

Second, today's Western culture places tremendous value on a genetically impossible-to-attain ideal of thinness for 98% of females. Third, the diet, entertainment, and fashion industries either market or perpetuate this impossible 'ideal' body as though everyone could easily attain it — if they are simply willing to spend their money on the advertised products and services — or at least make it look like they were getting there. Finally, adolescents live in a highly competitive and demanding society, where they can easily feel that doing their personal best still isn't good enough unless it meets some artificial, yet socially desired, standard of success and achievement.

All of these factors send several powerful messages to adolescents: significant and permanent weight loss is desirable, necessary, and possible; achieving thinness brings about a host of socially desirable rewards (e.g., success in all things, positive attention, sexual attractiveness, and a general state of happiness); achieving thinness or weight loss signals to others that you possess a unique capacity for self-discipline, mastery over your physical and emotional needs, and a 'specialness' that transcends any envied status in occupation, education, or wealth.

The eating disorder promises that everything else in your world will start to become okay, if not totally terrific, if you

You Can Help...

Let your son or daughter know that you are trying to understand and work with their hidden fears and resistance, while simultaneously ensuring that they are kept physically safe. Make sure they feel that you will stick by them.

can at least work toward the cultural ideal of beauty. Sounds like some pretty good reasons to start messing with your eating, weight, and shape, doesn't it?

The Adolescent Factor

But that's not the whole story. Add to this the fact that these powerful messages are often first taken in by young people during adolescence, at a time when their sense of confidence, self-esteem, and place in the world can be sent for a serious loop.

Adolescence marks a period in human development that comes with the demand to work successfully through a variety of important psychological tasks. If adolescents get stuck with one or more of the developmental tasks of adolescence, then it makes perfect sense that they would keep trying out different strategies until they finds one that works. The pursuit of thinness and all that is promised to come with it may serve as an effective adaptive or coping strategy.

If changing body image is indeed a new coping strategy, then it becomes more understandable why young people with eating disorders wouldn't be too keen to give it up. Why would they even want to conquer what gives them a sense of control, security, and success? This is especially true if they believe that they have no other way of dealing with the challenges of daily life in a similarly successful way. Not to mention the fact that you will be asking them to give up the pursuit of the ideal body, as well as the respect and admiration of their all-important circle of friends.

Changing Mind-sets

The irony in this particular viewpoint is that it is usually only some time after your child's goal of attaining some minimal body weight and shape has been achieved that all of the social and personal payoffs for this so-called success — positive social attention, sense of attractiveness, and sense of personal power and control — start to slip way. Your child's mind-set begins to shift away from the illusory belief in disordered eating as an adaptive coping strategy to the reality of disordered eating as the path to illness and despair. This will be a disturbing revelation for your child, but necessary for any treatment program to be effective.

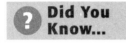

Did You Know...

• Despite numerous outward indicators of their actual success in the world, many young people with eating disorders silently carry the burden that they're still not good enough, not smart enough, not pretty enough, not popular enough, without talent, too big — ultimately, that they are somehow unlovable.

You Can Help...
Empathizing with your child's mind-set will send important messages that may have been drowned out during your battles to take away this central method of coping. Your willingness to consider another way of thinking about your child's eating disorder is a major step toward making an important therapeutic connection with your child. This connection will become especially apparent when your child starts to make changes leading toward active recovery.

Encouraging Change

Changing mind-sets about eating disorders tends to go hand in hand with different approaches to change. There is usually another discrepancy between parents and their children that tends to stall recovery and create loads of tension within the family. The child may not be ready to change.

Your task is to encourage change, educate where appropriate, and support your son or daughter as they discover their own readiness to change. If you force change, by pushing too hard or too early, your best intentions may make your child feel worse.

What other choice is there? You can meet your son or daughter at their level. You don't have to agree with their pursuit of thinness and eating disorder attitudes, but you could try to engage them in a way that helps them to feel 'heard' and not dismissed as "talking crazy" or "being irrational."

By now, your child may be sensitive to everything you say, waiting for you to say something that pushes the 'buttons' once again. Avoid a battle of wills by validating your child's views. This type of interaction can only lead to a win-win situation. While this is not a treatment or a cure for the eating disorder, this kind of relationship lowers parent-child tension and invites your child to confide in you while exploring the possibility of making changes.

Stages of Change

Researchers in the area of behavioral psychology have shown that people change their health behavior by progressing through a sequence of six motivational stages: precontemplation, contemplation, preparation, action, maintenance, and termination. This theory has been established for numerous health-related and addictive behaviors, such as smoking, alcohol and drug use, safe-sex practices, and cardiac care.

Applying specific strategies for change at specific stages of change is proving to be the most effective approach for maximizing psychological and behavioral change.

That you are reading this book to find help for your child's disordered eating is a sign that you are already beyond the precontemplation and contemplation stages, in preparation for the action stage of change. Your child is most likely to be in the precontemplation stage.

Here are the six stages of change, with the corresponding attitude of a child or adolescent with an eating disorder.

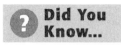

Did You Know...

● If young people are helped to progress from a stage of precontemplation (resisting change to a stage of contemplation (thinking about changing) within a month, then they will be twice as likely to take effective, self-directed action toward their own recovery over the next 6 months.

1. Precontemplation (Resisting Change)

The young person does not believe there is a problem. "I'm only here because someone else thinks I have an eating problem."

2. Contemplation (Thinking about Change)

The young person begins to accept the possibility of having an eating disorder. "I may have an eating disorder, but I'm not sure I can or want to change."

3. Preparation (Planning to Change)

The young person starts to get ready to make changes by considering the pros and cons of living with the eating disorder. "I'm planning to do something about my eating disorder really soon. I've started to explore and discuss what to do."

4. Action (Changing)

The young person takes active steps toward changing eating behaviors and thoughts. "I have been actively trying to do things to recover from my eating disorder."

5. Maintenance (Maintaining Changes)

The young person has made these changes but continues to be aware of the eating disorder. "I have made changes to solve my eating disorder but need to maintain these changes actively."

6. Termination (Moving On)

The young person has incorporated these changes into everyday life and the eating disorder is no longer an issue. "I am enjoying a normal, healthy lifestyle."

HELP FOR ENCOURAGING CHANGE

Do	Don't
Express concern about the problem behavior.	Nag!
Encourage your child to think about change.	Push your child into action.
Show your belief that things can be changed.	Give up on your child.
Address specific disruptive and distressing behaviors.	Pretend that a problem does not exist.
Insist that your son or daughter take responsibility for their actions.	Make excuses, cover up for, or defend the problem behavior.
Recognize that feeling down and discouraged some of the time is normal.	Expect your child to always feel positive.
Care for your child unconditionally.	Place conditions on your support.
Help your child identify what triggers problem behaviors.	Criticize your child for the problem behavior.
Talk to your child about the day's happenings and any special accomplishments or interests.	Keep asking your son or daughter how they are doing.
Offer to support anything they may do that shows a desire to change.	Expect your daughter or son to change all by themselves.
Show confidence in your child's ability to change.	Feel sorry for your child.
Review this list with your daughter or son.	Discuss this chart without your child's participation.

Phases of Recovery

Once your child shows a willingness to change, the most frequently asked question that parents have is: "How long will it take for my child to get better?" This is a difficult question to answer because there are just as many possible pathways 'out' of an eating disorder as there are possible pathways 'into' an eating disorder. Each child with an eating disorder and each family has a unique history and set of circumstances.

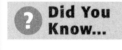

? Did You Know...

● Recovery from an eating disorder can be seen to progress through four phases: onset, discovery, resistance, and cooperation.

While questions about the course of the illness are therefore very individual, recovery from an eating disorder tends to fall into four phases that have been charted in clinical research and confirmed by clinical experience.

A review of these phases shows what you can expect to encounter as you help your child work toward recovery. It's not only *what* you do to try to help your child, but *when* you do it that is also important. The timing of the treatment strategy should complement the specific stage of your child's illness. This understanding will go a long way to improve the chances of recovery and minimize conflict.

Phase I: Onset

During the onset phase of an eating disorder, the young person's physical and psychological health diverge. While they may think they are feeling better psychologically because of their new eating behavior, they are beginning to suffer physically. The psychological line moves upward, as young people feel better about themselves and describe themselves as "doing well." (See the graph, "Four Phases of an Eating Disorder.") The physical line moves downward, however, as their bodies fall below their healthy weight and the eating disorder begins to have a subtle negative impact on physical functioning.

Psychological High

During onset, young people identify the eating disorder as an effective strategy for coping with the trials of adolescence. From their point of view, what's not to like about this? "I'm losing weight, feeling better, feeling happier. I'm being told that I look great, I'm feeling a sense of control and personal power, and, get this — I've also found a way to drive my parents crazy, get their attention, and get them to treat me

FOUR PHASES OF AN EATING DISORDER

This graph shows two lines that represent the psychological and physical functioning of an adolescent with anorexia nervosa from the beginning of disordered eating through to recovery. Before the onset of the disorder, the psychological and physical lines were quite close together, indicating that the child felt okay physically and psychologically. During onset, the lines diverge radically, alternate during discovery and resistance, and then coincide again during cooperative recovery.

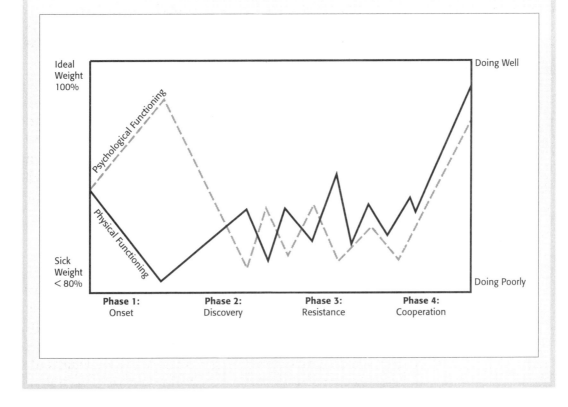

differently — and usually in a way that suits me better. Sounds like a plan!"

As they become thinner and thinner, they are rewarded for their control over their hunger by feeling psychologically stronger and more confident. They may also be rewarded for the obvious change in physical appearance through positive comments that initially come from friends and family, such as "You're looking well" or "You look so good, you've lost so much weight!" When you ask your child if anything is wrong, you will be reassured, "Everything is fine, not to worry, just leave me alone."

Physical Low

Behind this apparently happy and confident voice is another one telling them they are fat, ugly, unlikable, useless, and unlovable, and always will be — *unless* they pay close attention and start to restrict their eating, lose weight, and ignore the advice of others. If they follow along, then the voice of the eating disorder promises that all the negatives in their life will lift and that they will arrive at a much happier place. The voice of the eating disorder may add, "But you can't share our plan with anyone. They won't understand and will try to take away what you are working so hard to win for yourself."

Your child's real voice, while still present, has become quieter. A healthy voice is still trying to remind your son or daughter that they need to eat in order to stay healthy, that losing too much weight isn't good, that they are getting sick and will get sicker if they don't start to eat better.

As the eating disorder starts to get a stronger hold on your child, the eating disorder voice will try to drown out both you and your child's healthy voice.

You Can Help...

Let your daughter or son know that you are sensitive to the fact that they aren't just battling you about what eating well and being healthy means, but they are also battling an intrusive, highly manipulative, very convincing, yet destructive voice of an eating disorder.

Phase II: Discovery

For parents, the next phase of the eating disorder begins when they realize: "That's enough! This has to stop!" For adolescents (and their eating disorder voice), this is the moment when they realize: "We're busted! The secret's out!"

In the discovery phase, the eating disorder is confronted, first by you, then by your doctor, and at last by your child. If the eating disorder hasn't yet taken a firm hold, there is a very good chance your child will advance quickly through Phase II and III and be well on the way to recovery.

Once the eating disorder behaviors and beliefs are discovered, appropriate interventions should begin as soon as possible. These treatments will certainly include the restoration of a healthy weight, which may involve hospitalization, depending on the severity of the disorder.

Eating Therapy

You and your doctor should encourage your child to start eating again and to reduce the intensity and frequency of any methods of weight control being used. Their eating will likely remain problematic throughout this phase as they struggle to rediscover what foods they used to like eating and to reconnect with the non-dieting lifestyle they had prior to the onset of their eating disorder.

8 STEPS TO EATING HEALTHY AGAIN

There are eight key strategies for getting a child with an eating disorder to eat again.

1. Create clear expectations for eating and weight gain.

2. Set up valued rewards and enforce consequences linked to eating and weight gain.

3. Be upfront, truthful, predictable, and consistent in all interactions.

4. Acknowledge how difficult, confusing, or painful these changes can be.

5. Establish a safe emotional environment where all feelings can be expressed and where there is no fear that your child or anyone else will be allowed to lose control.

6. Assure your son or daughter that it is part of your job as a caring parent to not let them become physically sick in any way.

7. Always work with or talk directly to the 'healthy voice' that exists within your child (literally telling them that you don't want to speak to their eating disorder, but are now talking to the healthy person).

8. Let your child know that there are other, non-eating disordered ways of achieving personal success and happiness, and that you are ready to help your child discover and pursue them.

Physical Highs, Psychological Lows

Your child will begin to show some improvements in physical and nutritional health that will be very encouraging to you, but rather distressing to your child. There may be some deterioration in the previously positive psychological frame of mind, since it was deceivingly based on the eating disorder's illusion of feeling better and doing well. This decline in psychological functioning is usually seen as an increase in the young person's emotional and behavioral expression of anxiety, irritability, and moodiness.

Hospitalization for treatment of the disorder will provoke different responses. Inpatient units may help to motivate young people to change. There may be a genuine desire to change expressed upon being admitted to an inpatient unit as they recognize the consequences of their worsening eating problems.

However, the change in behavior may be deceptive. Some adolescents will say and do anything that they believe will get you and everyone else off their backs so that they can return to their original pursuit of thinness — including a begrudging willingness to eat and gain just enough weight to get themselves discharged from their treatment program. Keep in mind that it is the eating disorder that is manipulative and sneaky here.

CASE STUDY Brad

Some days, Brad's mother thought that she was going crazy…was it because she was exhausted from her pregnancy or worn out from the day-to-day challenges with Brad?

She contacted the family therapist on the eating disorder team to get some help with her struggle. The therapist was supportive. At first he just listened, then they identified what was going on, and finally they discussed how to address the issues. The therapist suggested that she had to work on understanding what Brad was going through.

Brad's mother decided to talk with him. She made sure to do less talking and more listening. She realized that growing up was especially hard for a sensitive and cautious boy like her son. Brad was a child who wanted to get everything right, including his body weight, shape, and size. He worried about making mistakes. He worried about being liked. It seemed like everything made him anxious.

Brad's mom tried to imagine what it would be like to live in her son's head. She felt exhausted. Listening really helped Brad's mom to understand what he was thinking. She no longer felt as frustrated by his struggle.

continued on page 160

> ## You Can Help...
> If the eating disorder voice has had the time to make its case for the pursuit of thinness, your child will likely fight to keep the eating disorder. You need to help your daughter or son find the strength to fight back, with you at their side.

Phase III: Resistance

In the resistance phase, children and adolescents with eating disorders often begin to cooperate but then react with intense negative emotions, such as anger, defiance, and paranoia. These emotions will rock the entire family. Because hope is often built up and then dashed and because these emotions are so intense, this is the most difficult phase of the illness.

Feeling Worse, Becoming Better

The psychological health of young people with eating disorders now falls below their (improved) level of physical health. They often need to feel worse before they can start to feel better. In this case, feeling worse usually refers to feeling worse emotionally and acting out according to the current sense of distress. From a positive perspective, the fact that your child has entered this more intense phase of the illness is a good sign because it usually signals a significant move toward recovery.

The nature of the effort that is required by your child and your family in this phase is best described by the saying that "the only way *out* is *through*." In order for your child to get 'out' of the eating disorder, both you and your child need to go 'through' or work 'through' whatever physical, psychological, emotional, or family-related issues are distressing your child and leading your child, paradoxically, to find comfort in an eating disorder.

Ways to Be

During this tense period, there are two basic ways for you 'to be' with your child — you will need to be patient and you will need to persevere.

You need to be patient while you put up with this intense expression of negative emotions, maintaining your composure and compassion when faced with unjustified outbursts and often hurtful comments about everything from your personal values and mental competency to your capacity to be a caring and trustworthy parent. You will need to try to remain calm and supportive in the face of these irrational patterns of behavior. Remind yourself, this is a necessary phase in recovery and may be linked to the numerous psychological tasks and challenges that are part of normal adolescent development.

A second 'way to be' is to persevere in your efforts to help your child gain control over the eating disorder. You will need to find your own comfort zone and set your own rules as to what is and what is not considered acceptable conduct within your family. This may be the time for you to adopt a 'parents know what's best for their child' stance to counteract any insurgence from the eating disorder voice. You will need to assert your voice, making it clear that you have real authority — it is your job to set and enforce the family rules with reasonable input from others.

By now, the eating disorder voice has given your child a tremendous capacity to defy your rules, to test your limits, and to endure your disciplinary actions. Unsuspecting parents and families can be worn down by the eating disorder's anger, defiance, resistance, and endurance. The eating disorder tries to keep pushing until the family either gives in or gives up in a state of total frustration and emotional exhaustion. You will need to stand fast against this assault.

You Can Help...

Try applying the four "Ways of Being with Your Child" to manage other teenage behaviors or attitudes within this stage. You should eventually notice their eating patterns starting to improve and their severest moods beginning to mellow. You allowed the eating disorder voice to have its tantrum, but also created the psychological space for your child to work things out and the freedom to choose a better way of being. The payoff is that these changes are a very encouraging sign of your child's chances of moving toward recovery.

WAYS OF BEING WITH YOUR CHILD
Motivational Interviewing

A very successful therapeutic 'way of being' with your child comes from an approach called motivational interviewing. The four general principles for this way of interacting with your child are well worth some experimentation. Be consistent and be patient.

1. Express Empathy and Your Belief in Your Child

- I will let her know that I am *trying* to understand her unique situation, her feelings and her motives. (She may not believe me if I say that I already truly understand her.)
- I will let him know that I believe in him and that I value his attempts to work things out for himself.
- I must choose to believe that my acceptance of my daughter helps her to grow and facilitates change, especially when the going gets tough.
- When he seems to want to talk, I must stop whatever I'm doing and really listen to him. When he's finished saying what he has to say, I can show him I've listened by summarizing it back to him.
- I need to live my life knowing that my daughter's ambivalence is normal – for both the eating disorder and for being a teenager.

2. Work through Resistance

- He is often going to meet new ideas, suggestions, and activities with resistance. I will try not to oppose his resistance directly. Instead, I will try to roll with his resistance and rejection, by finding the positives in no change and encouraging him to be the one who tells me that he is struggling with something that he is considering changing.
- I will avoid arguing for change – which usually gets me nowhere anyway. Instead, I can let her know that I believe that she is her own best resource for finding her own answers and solutions. If she says she's not, I will ask permission to try and help her.

3. See from the Outside-In and the Inside-Out

- I will help my daughter to talk about her personal goals and the things she dreams will make for a happy life.
- I can help him to become aware of the disagreement between his present attitude or behaviors and his personal goals and values that he shares with me.
- I will ask her to tell to me what she thinks I'm thinking. I will have her tell me what she thinks other people think about her when she does or says this or that.
- I will help my son to discover and present his own arguments for making change.

4. Create Optimism

- I will encourage my son's belief in the possibility of change and hope for the future.
- I will encourage my daughter's belief in her ability to make the changes.
- I will let her know that I am here to help, but that it is her responsibility to make changes herself.
- My belief in my child becomes a self-fulfilling prophecy.

The Way Through

Trying to reason with an eating disorder will never work because the very nature of the eating disorder is irrational, illogical, and self-destructive. You need to accept this and move on to doing whatever it takes to keep your child physically and psychologically healthy.

Treatment programs do not try to convince your daughter or son that their eating disorder is bad for them before they provide life-sustaining treatment. The trickiest part for parents is knowing how to balance their appreciation of their children's suffering and their desire to respect their psychological needs with their awareness that they need to do whatever they can to keep their child out of physical danger. Part of the solution is for parents to know that it is both expected and necessary for things to heat up while the eating disorder runs itself into the ground. Only then will the healthy voice of your child re-emerge.

Be sure to provide your child with support and compassion, despite the fact that your son or daughter may temporarily regress to an earlier level of disordered eating and emotional isolation. Help them to regain control and take responsibility for their own behavior. Remember, the only way 'out' is 'through.'

Phase IV: Cooperation

In the cooperation phase, both the physical and psychological lines of recovery now begin a steady rise toward a healthy weight and a healthy mind-set.

As young people with eating disorders begin to recognize that their sense of self and their personal success are not necessarily connected to body image, weight, and shape, they will move into the final phase of recovery. During this period, they choose to listen to their own voice over the now dulled eating disorder voice. They also begin to listen to *your* voice. They come to understand that you have not lied to them, never misled them, always believed in them, and steadfastly guided them with love.

They will start to eat more normally with less fear at every mouthful. They will be willing to take increasingly larger risks with previously forbidden foods. They will be ready to experiment with the timing of meals and snacks.

They will also reconnect with old friends and show increasing interest in teenage activities. They will show that they are learning to handle intense feelings more independently and to express their strong feelings more appropriately.

They will begin to work with their parents in a truly cooperative fashion to make changes in their lives and to maintain these changes.

In a perfect world, the cooperation phase would come to an end and your child would be completely free of the eating disorder. Given the realities of our present body-image-obsessed society, some disordered attitudes and feelings may linger, but they will remain inactive as the changes in behavior are maintained. Like many young people who have never had an eating disorder, your child will be conscious of body weight, shape and size issues, but will choose to continue living a healthy life.

TWO TAOIST PRINCIPLES

Resist with Nonresistance

One way for parents to counter the eating disorder voice is through a form of nonresistance practiced in the martial arts. Judo and jujitsu apply a method for winning a battle that capitalizes on the principle of not resisting your attacker. Through the clever redirection of the attacker's own weight and strength, the defender invites continued attacks, knowing that the attacker will eventually become exhausted. This is achieved without any aggressive counterattack. Resist with nonresistance. Attackers will see that their current approach won't succeed and concede to their opponent.

"To win 100 victories in 100 battles is not the highest skill," Chinese philosopher Sun Tzu said. "To subdue the enemy without fighting is the highest skill." Or as karate master Tsutomu Oshima said, "In order to achieve victory you must place yourself in your opponent's skin. If you don't understand yourself, you will lose 100% of the time. If you understand yourself, you will win 50% of the time. If you understand yourself and your opponent, you will win 100% of the time." By understanding the nature of the eating disorder afflicting your child, you will have a much better chance of victory.

Going with the Flow

Another principle of judo and jujitsu is to live within the flow of things. A Taoist story tells of an old man who accidentally fell into the river rapids leading to a high and dangerous waterfall. Onlookers feared for his life. Miraculously, he came out alive and unharmed downstream at the bottom of the falls. People asked him how he managed to survive. "I accommodated myself to the water, not the water to me. Without thinking, I allowed myself to be shaped by it. Plunging into the swirl, I came out with the swirl. This is how I survived."

PREPARING FOR THE JOURNEY

To prepare for the potentially long and hard road to recovery, consider the following advice from health-care professionals and fellow parents of children with eating disorders.

Don't

- Don't try to reason or argue with your child's eating disorder. You will be fruitlessly trying to reason with a relentless illness that is deceptive, irrational, and highly manipulative.

- Don't allow young people with eating disorders to make decisions about their eating (and perhaps everything else) with the false belief that they simply have to discover the error of their ways, after which they will simply snap out of it. They won't.

Do

- Do educate yourself about the nature and the treatments for eating disorders. Try to interest your child in understanding more about their eating, weight, and body image concerns.

- Do try out various behavioral change strategies that either reward good eating efforts or establish consequences for refusing to eat or for continuing with dangerous weight control methods.

Prospects for Recovery

Research has shown that four main factors influence the outcome of any therapy for eating disorders. Some factors have a greater influence than others, as shown here in the percentile ranking.

1. Patient Characteristics (40%)

The patient is verbal or talkative, insightful, open to new ideas and behaviors, willing to experiment with change, willing to risk new ways of thinking about family functioning, values, and culture.

2. Therapist Characteristics (30%)

The therapist is not only an expert but empathic, warm, supportive, and nonjudgmental. The patient trusts the therapist.

3. Type and Timing of Therapy (15%)

The right type of therapy is administered at the right time in the recovery process. At one stage, a particular strategy or therapy may turn out to be a miserable failure, but at another stage, the same approach may prove to be highly successful.

4. Patient's Hope and Belief in the Process (15%)
The patient has confidence in the therapy process.

Parent's Role

As a parent, your job is to create the winning conditions for your child's recovery by establishing a relationship with your child that is characterized by trust, warmth, empathy, and support, not ambivalence, conflict, inconsistency, or uncertainty. If you and your child can create some belief in each other and develop confidence that you'll get through this, you will have done a significant portion of the therapeutic work necessary for a good psychological outcome. With your support, guidance, and love, your child can become healthy again.

CASE STUDY Jessica

After my initial visit to the 'diet' doctor, I let my parents know that I hadn't lost any weight. My parents got really angry. They had spent good money to help me lose weight. All the way home in the car we said horrible things to one another. I accused them of not loving me because I was "too fat" to be loved. When we got home, I ran upstairs and the first thing I did was binge. I had some food stashed away for this kind of situation. At times like this, it seemed like only binging would help me feel better. I would worry about the consequences later.

A few hours later, my dad knocked on my bedroom door and came in. The first thing he did was to apologize. Then he started telling me what it was like for him being fat while growing up and how horribly he was treated by others. He wanted me to lose weight so that I wouldn't have to experience the same torment and humiliation that he endured.

For the first time, in as long as I can remember, my dad and I talked. I told him everything that was going on with my eating and my binging. He just listened…he really listened and it felt good. Finally, in my dad's sympathetic and thoughtful way, he suggested that I needed to get some help to assist me in feeling better about myself. He assured me that he and my mom would help me figure out what we needed to do. He asked me if I would work with them on moving forward with this plan. I jumped at the chance!

continued on page 211

CHAPTER 10

Exploring Treatment Resources in Your Community

Navigating the health-care system and achieving the best care possible for your child can be a challenge at the best of times. This can be particularly demanding when your child has an eating disorder. Parents know when their child is sick, but often struggle with finding the treatment they need.

Trying to figure out what you can do to help your child can be a daunting task. In many communities, the treatment for children and adolescents with eating disorders is quite limited. It is not unusual for health-care professionals to have little knowledge about eating disorders. Finding treatment for your child can feel next to impossible. Knowing how to access all resources in your own community for treating your child is, therefore, vitally important.

Where Do We Start?

Don't despair! There are resources available for children and adolescents who suffer from an eating disorder.

Family Doctor or Pediatrician

The first and most important resource is your family physician or pediatrician. If you think your child is having problems with eating, talk to your doctor. Do not hesitate to call right away if you are worried about your child. Make the time to talk with your doctor by telephone.

COMMUNITY RESOURCES CHECKLIST

This checklist provides a progressive guide to finding resources in your health-care community for treating your child with an eating disorder. Plan your exploration with this list and check off each possibility once you have gathered the information you need.

Resource

☐ Contact your family doctor or pediatrician to make an appointment for an assessment.

☐ Gather information on eating disorder services in the community.

☐ Review eating disorder information with your doctor.

☐ In partnership with your doctor or other knowledgeable health-care professional, select an appropriate eating disorder treatment resource.

☐ Contact local social service agencies regarding additional support (travel, accommodation, child care, etc.)

☐ Arrange for your doctor to monitor your child while you are awaiting further service.

☐ Follow the recommended treatment plan from the eating disorder service.

When it comes to the medical care for your child, your doctor knows your child's health history best. He should have your child's medical records and the most up-to-date information on your child's health. If you have changed doctors, be sure to have your child's medical records transferred to your new doctor. The more complete your medical records are, the better informed your doctor will be.

Most likely, your doctor will have knowledge about child and adolescent eating disorders. Your doctor will be able to refer you to other resources in the health-care community. Some family physicians and pediatricians may have additional training in this area.

Specialized Services

Getting your child's health care from someone other than your own doctor outside your local community may be overwhelming. Lack of proximity to treatment centers offers many challenges.

Q: What will happen when I contact my child's doctor?

A: When you call your doctor, have a pen and paper ready to write down any instructions, advice, and questions. It is easy to forget some details, especially when you are worried about your child. Don't be disappointed or surprised if your doctor is not able to answer your questions without seeing your child first.

You and your child may need to make an appointment to discuss your concerns face-to-face. After this initial meeting, your doctor may inform you that your child is, in fact, suffering with an eating disorder and should be closely monitored over the next few months. Your doctor may find the eating disorder to be more severe and refer you immediately to a pediatrician specializing in eating disorders or to a specialized eating disorder program.

Generally speaking, specialized eating disorder services, especially those for children and adolescents, are more likely to be found in larger cities than in rural communities. If you live in a rural community and your doctor refers you to a center that offers specialized eating disorder services, you may need to travel a long distance to receive treatment for your child.

FACTORS INFLUENCING REFERRALS TO EATING DISORDER SPECIALISTS

There are a number of factors that you and your doctor will need to consider when looking for appropriate services to treat your child's eating disorder.

- Where you live and how close you are to pediatric health-care professionals or specialized pediatric eating disorder services.

- What types of services your child and family need and are available in your community.

- The age and development of your child.

- Your willingness and your child's willingness to participate in treatment.

- Cost of service and your ability to afford the service.

To make this more manageable, many families choose to work with both their local health-care professionals with support from specialized eating disorder services elsewhere. Specialized services often welcome the opportunity to collaborate with local community health centers, where they provide training, consultations, and clinical support as required. Work with your doctor to find local services that can be put together to help treat your child or adolescent. For instance, there may be a dietitian in your community who can work with your doctor to treat your child. In such circumstances, families may still need to travel to the specialized treatment centers, but much less frequently.

Keep in mind that there are various approaches to eating disorder assessments and treatment. Find or create an option that is comfortable and effective for your needs. No one approach is superior to another.

Q: How long will we have to wait before seeing a specialist?

A: Some eating disorder services are able to provide immediate assessments, while others may have a lengthy waiting period. Ask your doctor how long the waiting period might be. Regardless, it is important to have your child followed regularly by your doctor until such time.

If you feel that your child is getting worse, then you should contact your doctor immediately. If your doctor is concerned that your child is getting worse, then your doctor should contact the specialized services earlier.

Moreover, if your child seems to be improving, don't immediately assume that your child has recovered. Children and adolescents with eating disorders usually take months to years to recover. Therefore, continue to see your doctor regularly until you are both confident that your child is no longer struggling with the eating disorder. This should be a decision that both the family and the doctor make together.

A DOZEN QUESTIONS TO ASK ABOUT EATING DISORDER SERVICES

When you contact health-care professionals offering specialized eating disorder services, you should interview them. Have your questions written down ahead of time so you don't forget them. Write down the answers and make sure you understand them. If there is information you don't understand, ask for an explanation. You might want to take another adult with you. It is often better to have more than one person hearing all the information.

The following is a list of questions you might want to ask when contacting an eating disorder service. For that matter, these questions apply to a family doctor, pediatrician, psychiatrist, individual therapist, social worker, psychologist, dietitian, or any combination of treatment professionals. Don't be afraid to ask your questions or ask where you can find more information.

1. What is your basic approach to treatment?

Get a sense of the health-care professional's basic approach to treatment well in advance of your assessment. Work toward a good understanding of how much the health-care professionals and you agree on the proposed treatment. Ask them to describe treatment options thoroughly. If you are unsure about these options, review them with your family doctor or pediatrician.

Notes:

_____

_____

_____

_____

2. What kind of information do you need before you assess our child and family?

You need to prepare your child, other family members, and yourself for the assessment process. You will also want to ensure that your doctor will be monitoring your child while you wait for the assessment and the development of a treatment plan.

Notes:

_____

_____

_____

_____

_____

_____

3. Who are the health-care professionals who will be meeting with my child and our family?

The composition of the assessment team will vary depending on the particular health-care setting. In some situations, an assessment will be completed by a team of health-care professionals from many different disciplines, such as a pediatrician or family doctor, a dietitian, a child psychiatrist, a nurse, a psychologist, and a social worker. Other assessment teams may have one to three disciplines. You will want to know how experienced these people are in treating pediatric eating disorders. Reassure yourself that the treatment team is well-qualified to help.

Notes: _____

_____

_____

_____

4. What if my child or family does not speak or understand English easily?

You will want to explore the availability of an interpreter in this case.

Notes: _____

_____

_____

_____

5. Will you need to meet with our family?

You will need to know what role your family will play in the assessment and treatment process, what commitments this will involve, when and where. Does the clinic have flexible hours or offer after-school, early morning, weekend, or evening appointments?

Notes: _____

_____

_____

_____

_____

_____

_____

_____

WORKSHEET

6. How long do the appointments last?

You will need to plan your time as well so you can make arrangements at work or for care of your other children. Knowing how long an appointment may last will also help you to prepare your child for the event.

Notes:

_____

_____

_____

7. How will the health-care professionals communicate with our family doctor or pediatrician about the ongoing treatment?

You will want to see a clear plan of collaboration between the eating order specialists and your doctor during treatment and in planning ongoing care after treatment.

Notes:

_____

_____

_____

8. What if we have questions?

Establishing your key contact at the clinic is important. You will want to speak to this person on a regular basis as new questions arise, when you need to confide information, and when you need further help. You may want to know if you can contact this person outside of scheduled appointments.

Notes:

_____

_____

_____

9. What if our child has questions?

Again, you will want your child to feel comfortable in confiding with one of the treatment team members and asking them questions.

Notes:

_____

_____

_____

_____

_____

_____

WORKSHEET

10. Do I have to pay for the services provided by the health-care professionals or treatment facility?

You will need to know if your private or public health-care plan covers the costs of assessment and treatment. Review what services are and are not included in your insurance policy and to what extent they are reimbursable. Health-care professionals may be able to tailor a treatment program that suits your child and is covered under your insurance policy. For services that might not be covered by your insurance policy, they may also be able to advise you if there is a special fee schedule or sliding scale fee to accommodate various financial circumstances. There may be other sources of financial support they can draw on.

Notes: _____

_____

_____

11. What if we have to travel a long distance to come to the treatment center...are we eligible for assistance with travel expenses?

Your family may be eligible for assistance with travel expenses. Contact your local social service agencies to inquire. If you have to travel a long distance to obtain specialized eating disorder services, this support may help with the travel and accommodation costs. Many countries have social service agencies that will work with your family to provide additional support for these expenses.

Notes: _____

_____

_____

12. Do you have any services that parents and siblings can access for help?

You will want to know what support groups may be available and suitable for your personal needs as parents and for your other children. Most eating disorder services and clinics are most willing to help parents and siblings of the child with an eating disorder. You are instrumental in the recovery of your child.

Notes: _____

_____

_____

_____

Where Do We Find Good Information?

When a family has a child with an eating disorder, there will be no end to the advice you receive from well-meaning and caring people. Your friends, extended family members, television, movies, books, newspapers, the Internet, community members, work acquaintances, and many more will all have ideas about what you should do.

The best way to seek out an appropriate assessment and treatment is to take the time to gather information from reliable sources. Never hesitate to speak directly with your doctor or other knowledgeable health-care professionals to discuss the information you have gathered. Then, plan accordingly. It is important to try to understand the struggles that your son or daughter is facing, but don't let these difficulties stop you from doing what is in their best interest. Never be afraid to ask questions or ask for a second opinion. The only way to understand a program fully and what it has to offer is to ask questions…many questions.

Q: We have found an eating disorder program that we think would be effective for our child and family. How do we seek their help?

A: If you have found a resource that you believe is appropriate for you and your child, there are several ways to access these services. Some services allow for self-referral, which means you or your child can call the program directly and make an appointment for an assessment. Other services may require a referral from your doctor or other health-care professional.

Your doctor may need to call or write a letter requesting that your child have an assessment. In some cases, the referring doctor may be asked to complete a referral form that provides information about your child's current illness and past medical health, including your child's previous growth and development, growth curves, psychiatric history, and family history. Your doctor may need to re-evaluate your child in order to provide current medical information to complete this form.

CASE STUDY Martha

Martha loved surfing the web. One evening she was bored and keyed in the word "bulimia." She was amazed at what came up. She found a website that was developed by a person with bulimia nervosa. This website had a few links that led her to a chat room where she could talk to other people who seemed to understand her.

Bulimia nervosa made sense for the people in the chat-room. Everyone treated bulimia like a good friend. They called bulimia "Mia." Mia was their friend. The more Martha learned about Mia, the more she grew to like and depend on her. Mia took on a life of her own...she was almost like a real person. Her buli'MIA' became her best friend.

Martha went to the chat room frequently until one of her brothers caught her. They shared a computer. He had snooped in her address book. He went on some of the sites and was mortified when he read the information on these "pro-mia" websites. Martha's brother busted her. She was convinced he did this so he could have more computer time.

Unfortunately, they both suffered. The computer was moved to the family room just off the kitchen, where her parents could monitor her computer use. Although her brother also lost his privacy, he insisted it was okay if it would help Martha.

continued on page 175

Reliable Information

There are many sources of information on eating disorders. Evaluate these resources critically in order to protect yourself and your child from the unhealthy information you read, watch, or hear. Your health-care professional can help you determine which messages are useful.

Internet

The Internet has become a frequently used resource for accessing information. It can be a useful tool to help find information and locate services for eating disorders in your community. However, it is advisable that you enlist the help of people who can tell the difference between accurate, useful information and inaccurate, harmful information. Evaluate the content of websites carefully. If you are not sure about the validity of the content, then check with your health-care professional. You might want to take a copy of the information with you to your next appointment so that you can discuss it with your doctor.

Advocacy Groups

Some eating disorder advocacy groups compile lists and databases with listings of health-care professionals and professional organizations that provide eating disorder treatment. Put together your own list of individuals or groups who provide treatment in your region. Speak to these individuals or groups directly to find out more about their services.

Many established eating disorder programs have written information or websites that include a description of the program, an overview of the staff members in the program, contact information, and a guide for accessing their service. In addition, they may also have information on the signs and symptoms, treatments, and new research findings for children suffering from eating disorders.

Community Information Centers

Often there is an information center in your library that may carry pamphlets or booklets about services available in your community. Community health groups, such as body-image coalitions, walk-in medical clinics, and community mental health clinics may also have information in the form of pamphlets, a reading list, or a directory of community resources on eating disorders. Staff at these facilities may also be a resource for families who are looking for services.

School teachers, guidance counselors, camp directors, religious leaders, or community service groups (Guides, Scouts, YMCA/YWCA) may have access to community supports and resources for children and adolescents who are in need of health services. Adults in these roles should also be aware of the signs and symptoms of eating disorders. These individuals may provide additional support to your child and may be able to help you or your child find appropriate resources.

Public Health Nurses

Public health nurses may have extensive information on services and resources in their local community. Some of these health-care professionals may have special knowledge of eating disorders services that may support your child and family.

Eating Disorder Books

Books on eating disorders, such as this one, often publish a list of resources. See the "Eating Disorders Information Resources" section in this book for more information on international, national, and regional eating disorder services.

? Did You Know...

• Well-established "pro-ana" and "pro-mia" websites are dedicated to showing young people how to be 'successful' anorexics or bulimics. They describe these eating disorders as a desirable lifestyle choice, not as a disease. They provide information on how best to starve and purge and how to keep these behaviors a secret.

• Monitor use of the Internet to ensure that your child is not enlisted on these sites.

KEY RESOURCES

There are central referral agencies in many countries where they keep an updated database on eating disorder treatment centers, agencies, and groups providing eating disorder services, as well as individual therapists and other professional groups offering support services.

Feel free to contact these agencies directly or discuss this list with your doctor to isolate the services best suited to your situation. Be sure to keep notes on what you discover. They may come in handy now as you arrange for the assessment and treatment of your child, or later if you decide to add or change treatment programs.

Provided here are the key resources with their websites. For a complete list of eating disorder resources, see the "Eating Disorder Information Resources" section of this book.

Academy for Eating Disorders (AED): www.aedweb.org.

American Academy of Child and Adolescent Psychiatry (AACAP): www.aacap.org

American Academy of Pediatrics (AAP): www.aap.org

American Dietetic Association (ADA): www.eatright.org

American Psychiatric Association (APA): www.psych.org.

Canadian Academy of Child and Adolescent Psychiatry: www.cnacad.org

Canadian Paediatric Society (CPS): www.caringforkids.cps.ca

Dietitians of Canada: www.dietitians.ca

Eating Disorder Referral and Information Center: www.EDReferral.com

Gurze Books: www.gurze.com

National Eating Disorder Information Centre (NEDIC): www.nedic.ca

National Eating Disorders Association (NEDA): www.edap.org

Society for Adolescent Medicine (SAM): www.adolescenthealth.org

Something Fishy: www.somethingfishy.org

Patience and Perseverance

Navigating the health-care system and accessing the best care possible for your child can take time and requires careful research. It is important to be proactive. Your family doctor and pediatrician are important resources for you and your child. Gather as much information as possible and review this with your doctor or health-care professional. They can help you with the many decisions that need to be made regarding your child. Don't hesitate to respond to what you feel may be a problem. By acting immediately, you can prevent an eating disorder from taking hold.

CHAPTER 11

Getting an Assessment

An eating disorder is a serious illness that requires professional intervention. Once this is recognized and your family has decided to seek treatment, the next step is getting an assessment of your child and your family. An eating disorder assessment is an important step on the road to recovery. The assessment is the foundation of a successful treatment program.

The decision to seek professional help for your child with an eating disorder is, however, a difficult one. Often the best way to begin is by arranging an appointment with your family doctor, pediatrician, or mental health-care professional. These people often know you and your family already. They will be able to advise you whether or not your child and family need a formal eating disorder assessment, and if so, will refer you to health-care professionals skilled in pediatric health, mental health, and eating disorders.

You Can Help...

Knowing what to expect from an assessment and how to prepare for one goes a long way in reducing any anxiety or fear you may feel. More importantly, if you are prepared for the assessment, you will be better able to support your child in preparing for this day. Although your child is the focus of the assessment, you can help the health-care professionals understand your child and the development of your child's eating disorder.

Parents are often as reluctant as their child to undergo an assessment, fearing that professionals will only confirm what they have come to believe — that they are inadequate parents. Parents often worry that they will be blamed for their child's eating disorder. Remember parents and teens are no more responsible for causing an eating disorder than they would be in causing other illnesses, such as diabetes or cancer. Many factors are involved in the development of an eating disorder, not just one. You may want to think about it as a collision of events that together lead up to the development of an eating disorder.

Although the waiting period to book an assessment is often filled with mixed feelings, once it has been arranged, family members will likely experience some relief.

To accomplish these objectives, health-care professionals need to understand all aspects of the child's functioning, now and in the past. They will also need to place this information in the context of the family and life environment. Identifying factors that may have precipitated the onset of the eating disorder and now perpetuate it is critical.

Q: Our family doctor has arranged for my son and our family to have an eating disorder assessment at the local children's hospital. I'm not so sure we need to follow through with this assessment because he seems to be gaining weight. He is insisting that he is better and doesn't need to go to this assessment. Do you think I should cancel this appointment?

A: One of the key issues in treating a child or adolescent with an eating disorder is dealing with their perceived sense of control. The desperate fear of being brought to treatment and losing all sense of self-control may lead them to plead with you to forgo the assessment.

This is often done in one of two ways. Some young people experience a 'temporary flight into health' and appear to make some significant, although transient, improvement. If this occurs, praise them for their success but insist that the assessment take place. Others become argumentative and rude or flaunt rules. Be sympathetic to their distress but remain firm. An eating disorder is a serious and often life-threatening chronic illness.

The good news is that the outcome of a child with an eating disorder is quite good, especially if your child is diagnosed, assessed, and treated early in the course of the illness.

ASSESSMENT OBJECTIVES

- To gather together a complete history of the development of the eating disorder.

- To arrive at a diagnosis.

- To determine the seriousness of the eating disorder.

- To learn about other situations in the child's life that may have an impact on the eating disorder.

- To develop a treatment plan.

The Assessment Team

An eating disorder is a chronic illness that not only causes serious medical problems but also affects a child's emotional and social well-being. In response to the medical, emotional, and social dimensions of eating disorders, a diverse group of health-care professionals usually conduct the assessment, though in some situations, an individual health-care professional with expertise in child and adolescent eating disorders may carry out the assessment. The assessment team is typically interdisciplinary, consisting of health-care professionals from many different disciplines, such as a pediatrician (often an adolescent medicine specialist) or family doctor, a child psychiatrist, a nurse, a psychologist, a dietitian, and a social worker.

You Can Help...

Parents are seen as active members of the assessment team. Your involvement is critical in gaining an understanding of your child and putting a treatment plan in place. Keep in mind that parents, more than anyone else, know their child best and are vital to helping members of the interdisciplinary team decide what may or may not work.

Preparing for the Assessment

After being referred for an assessment, you may have many questions to ask. Answering some of them here may make the prospect of the assessment less daunting for you and your child — and, ultimately, more successful for everyone involved.

Who Attends the Assessment?

Most settings request that both parents and their child be present at the initial assessment, with other family members included early on or at later stages of the treatment plan. With reconstituted families, the parent and step-parent with whom the child lives are usually asked to attend the initial assessment, while the other biological parent may be requested to attend or be asked to participate at a later date. In joint custody arrangements, the decision as to who should participate is best decided by both biological parents in conjunction with the advice of the assessment team. The assessment team will probably want to meet the affected child's siblings and stepsiblings at some point, although not necessarily at the first interview. Check this out in advance.

What Homework Can We Do?

In order to make best use of the time, the assessment team will request some background information. This may include information on previous assessments for this or other illnesses, previous hospitalizations, prior medical, psychiatric or psychological assessments, psychological tests, educational assessments, school evaluations, current or past medications, previous growth and weight charts, current or past laboratory studies, copies of previous EKG and X-ray studies. To this end, you and your child may be asked to fill out forms for the release of this confidential information to share with the assessment team. Getting these reports forwarded through the medical system is often a slow process, so you may want to pick up these reports yourself and deliver them to the assessment team before the first session or on the day of the assessment.

Be sure to keep a running list of questions or concerns that come up over the period prior to the assessment. This way, you are sure to get many of your questions answered.

> **? Did You Know...**
>
> • Studies have shown that when adolescents are assured confidential health care, they are more willing to disclose sensitive information about sexuality, substance use, and mental health.
>
> • They are also motivated to seek future health care.

Will the Assessment Be Confidential?

When your child and family are introduced to members of the assessment team, confidentiality should be discussed. The legal and ethical limitations of confidentiality will vary depending on the current laws in your province or state. Regardless, the adolescent should be made aware of the conditions under which confidentiality will be maintained. Examples of when confidentiality would not be upheld include situations when young people are at risk of hurting themselves or others. Under such circumstances, it would be necessary and appropriate for the health-care professional to inform the parents or guardians.

When young people have an opportunity to meet with a health-care professional on their own without their parents, they may feel more comfortable and less embarrassed to talk about difficult issues or humiliating behaviors. They do not have to worry about alarming their parents about these behaviors. Parents are not always aware of the extent of the eating problem or the magnitude of the unhealthy behaviors.

Confidential care for children and adolescents does not preclude the involvement of parents, however. In fact, medical research has shown that young people with eating disorders often freely share information with their parents, and this often occurs after they consult privately with their health-care professional. In the end, most children and adolescents will readily agree to allow their health-care professional to discuss the broad details of these issues with their parents.

Parents will often be given an opportunity to discuss any confidential issue they feel may not be appropriate to review in the presence of their child. Once again, the assessment team should review with the parents what the assessment team will keep confidential from their child.

How Will the Interviews Be Structured?

An assessment may take place all in one day or it may be scheduled in parts over several days or weeks. Different team members may take part in different stages of the assessment, though information will be shared between team members to reduce repetition as much as possible.

In some settings, selected members of the team (including trainees) will sit behind a one-way mirror and observe other members of the team carry out the assessment. This limits the number of people in the interview room and reduces the repetition of questions. Before using a one-way mirror, the team should inform you and your child and request your permission to do so.

Some settings may use a semi-structured interview, an informal, relaxed discussion based on broad pre-set questions that guide the discussion. These questions do not limit the conversation. The interviewer can ask new questions or elaborate on specific concerns as they arise. In a structured interview, the interviewer will stick to specific questions from a questionnaire or survey.

What Will Be the Outcome of the Assessment?

Keep in mind what an assessment will and will not offer your child and family. First, don't expect too much from the assessment; by itself, it won't solve the problem. The assessment will not determine the cause of the eating disorder. The assessment will not provide an immediate cure for the eating disorder. However, the assessment is the first step in getting your child treatment for the eating disorder. The assessment will help identify the problems that you and your child face. The assessment will set you and your child on the path to recovery.

COMPONENTS OF THE ASSESSMENT

These elements are common components of the assessment. Depending on the setting, they may be completed all at once or over time.

1. Medical assessment (medical history, physical examination, laboratory tests as required)

2. Family assessment (involving the child, the parents, and possibly the siblings)

3. Parent interview

4. Individual psychological assessment with the child

5. Complete nutritional history from the child and the family

6. Pencil and paper questionnaires completed by the patient and individual family members

---

Medical Examination

The pediatrician or family doctor will complete a medical history and physical examination as part of the eating disorder assessment.

Diagnosis

To confirm the diagnosis of an eating disorder, the doctor will rule out other possible medical and psychiatric causes of your child's behavior, including cancer, seizure disorders, inflammatory bowel disease, endocrine and metabolic disease, infection, and pregnancy. At the same time, the doctor will identify any coexisting medical conditions. Occasionally, eating disorders can occur simultaneously with other chronic illnesses, such as diabetes mellitus or Crohn's disease.

The doctor will establish the seriousness of the eating disorder in order to determine where (inpatient, outpatient, or day treatment) and how the child would be best treated. To prevent and treat the medical complications that so commonly occur with eating disorders, the doctor will continue to monitor your child's general health closely.

History

In order to accomplish this, the doctor must complete a thorough medical history. At first, the doctor will meet with you and your child together to establish why you have come for an assessment. This will allow the doctor to gather important information about your child's eating attitudes and behaviors. Together, you and your child will have an opportunity to express your thoughts and concerns. After you meet together, your child will have an opportunity to be interviewed alone. This part of the interview will include an account of the onset, duration, and course of the illness, as well as any previous treatments and results.

The doctor will also assess your child's satisfaction with body shape, weight, and size. Current eating patterns, behaviors, and means of weight control will be determined. Questions about vomiting, exercise (type, amount, frequency), and use of laxatives, diuretics, ipecac, diet pills, caffeine, and complementary and alternative medicines will be asked. Your doctor will also need to know if your child is taking any other medications, including thyroid medication, insulin, or oral contraceptives. Furthermore, the doctor will explore drug, alcohol, and tobacco use.

For your daughter, your doctor will complete a thorough menstrual history, asking if your daughter has started to menstruate and when she had her first menstrual period, as well as the length of her menstrual cycle, and the date and her weight at her last normal menstrual period.

Finally, as a part of any pediatric or adolescent assessment, the doctor may review your child's past physical and mental health and ask questions about how well other organ systems are working.

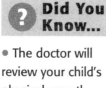

Did You Know...

• The doctor will review your child's physical growth and development, including your child's weight and height. This is when the previous growth charts are very helpful in understanding your child's growth and development.

Examination

A thorough physical examination is conducted because every organ system in the body can be affected by an eating disorder. The physical examination will help to identify any of the physical complications that can result from an eating disorder.

Your doctor will also determine your child's heart rate, breathing rate, blood pressure, and body temperature. The doctor will measure your child's current height and weight and compare it to previous heights and weights. This data will be plotted on a growth curve and compared to your child's earlier growth patterns. Your child's SMR will be documented. Then the doctor will examine every organ system in the body.

Tests

Laboratory tests can be helpful in making a diagnosis and identifying medical complications. No single laboratory test helps with the diagnosis; however, some blood tests will help rule out other medical conditions as well as complications of malnutrition.

Such blood tests might include a complete blood count (amount of red blood cells, white blood cells, and platelets in the body), electrolytes (minerals in the bloodstream), glucose, renal, liver, and thyroid function tests, amylase (an enzyme that occurs in the saliva and pancreas and helps with the digestion of starch; may be increased in young people who vomit), and other hormone tests. An EKG may be recommended, especially if your child has lost a great deal of weight, if your child is vomiting or using laxatives, diuretics, or ipecac, or if your child shows signs and symptoms of cardiac problems.

The doctor may suggest that a bone density test be done to assess the strength of your child's bones; low bone density is an early and potentially serious consequence of anorexia nervosa.

> **? Did You Know...**
>
> • A child's sexual maturity rating (SMR) is a way to document the physical progression of sexual maturation of breast and pubic hair development in females, and pubic hair, testicles, and penis development in males.
>
> • The SMR uses a 5-point scale. An SMR of 1 means that your daughter or son has not started puberty, whereas an SMR of 5 means that your daughter or son has reached full adult sexual maturation.

> **You Can Help...**
>
> Sometimes parents can do things differently to help their child fight the disorder. For example, in a family where the father suffers a heart attack and is prescribed a low-fat, low-cholesterol diet, his daughter may develop a belief that food containing fat will also place her at risk for heart disease. Uncovering such erroneous ideas and giving less attention to fat in the daily diet may help her to understand what eating behavior is appropriate for a healthy teenager.

Family Assessment

The goal of the family assessment is to gain some understanding of how the family works and how the eating disorder developed. It may include all family members living in your home or it may include the child with the eating problem and the parents or primary caregivers.

Different perspectives from various family members can help the treatment team to understand fully the issues and their impact on the child and the family. Teenagers will often minimize the extent of the problem, but hearing their parents talk openly about the problem will often increase their child's

ASSESSMENT INTERVIEW QUESTIONS

Be prepared and prepare your child — there will be many questions! Some are easy to answer; some can be difficult. For example:

Q: Describe who is in your family? Who lives in your home? Describe your strengths as a family?

Q: How do the members in your family get along?

Q: When did your child's problems with eating start?

Q: Who first noticed that there was a problem with your child's eating? What did they notice and what did they do?

Q: Tell me the story of your child's eating problems. Start from the beginning...

Q: Do you think that there was anything in particular that triggered the eating problems?

Q: What makes your child's eating problems better or worse?

Q: How does this affect you and your family?

Q: Is there anyone else in your family concerned about their weight, body shape, or size?

Q: Is there anyone in your family who has eating problems? Is there anyone in your family who has a mental illness, such as depression, anxiety, or obsessive-compulsive behavior?

Q: Does your family have meals together?

Q: How does your child do academically in school? How has your child done in the past? Any changes or concerns?

Q: How does your child interact socially? Have there been any recent changes in your child's friendships?

ability to speak more frankly about the disorder. The assessment team will observe how the child and parents interact on this issue, exploring each family member's past and current eating attitudes and behaviors. The family and the treatment team now begin to work together to solve the problem.

Parent Interview

During the parent interview, you will meet alone with the assessment team so they can further develop an understanding of your child, your family, and the eating disorder. Parents have an opportunity to speak about issues they feel may not be appropriate to discuss in the presence of their child. The parent interview provides a safe, adult space to talk more openly about these issues.

Many of the questions asked during the family interview will be repeated from the parents' perspective only. Parents will likely be asked about their own health, the health of their other children, and any psychiatric or emotional difficulties in family members, including your extended family. Now is a time for you to confide your own personal struggles in coping with your child's eating disorders. This interview is where you begin your relationship with the therapist.

You Can Help...

With your cooperation, the assessment team will complete a careful medical, developmental, and psychological history by asking about your child's developmental milestones and overall adjustment at different ages. You will be asked to identify concerns you have about your child's behavior, such as depressed mood, anxiety, school performance, and peer relationships. You may also be asked to discuss your relationship or couple issues that you may feel uncomfortable exploring in the presence of your child. For instance, there may be parental stresses or marital problems that may help your health-care professional understand your family better. Be sure to mention any challenges you are facing with the other children in your family.

Individual Interview

A child psychiatrist, psychologist, or social worker often conducts the individual interview with your child. During this session, the therapist will determine whether your son or daughter perceives that they have a problem and how they understand the problem.

Be forewarned — this interview may be difficult for your child. However, by the end of this interview, most young people experience relief. For the first time, they feel free to discuss issues they have often kept to themselves because they felt too embarrassed, humiliated, guilty, or sad to talk about them. The individual interview should help young people understand that they are not alone and that other teenagers suffer from similar problems. For many young people, it offers renewed hope of getting better.

Individual interviews usually start with open-ended questions. Your child may be asked, "Why have you come for an assessment?" The way a teenager answers this is often very informative. Some will say they have only come to this assessment because their parents insisted. In turn, they will insist that there is no problem, that their parents are overreacting. "Everything is under control," they will assert.

? Did You Know...

● More that half of all teenagers with eating disorders have other mental health problems. Your child should be carefully evaluated for signs and symptoms of depression, generalized anxiety, obsessive-compulsive symptoms, and previous traumatic experiences.

● Potential stresses, such as difficulties at school or problems with peers or family members, should also be explored.

Q: We have arranged an eating disorder assessment for our daughter. She has reluctantly agreed to go to the assessment but refuses to discuss "anything" with anyone! What should we do?

A: While you can force her to attend the assessment, you can't force her to participate and answer questions. Don't worry about this threat. Pediatric and mental health-care professionals are skilled at making children and adolescents feel at ease in difficult situations. They are trained to obtain information from children who may be reluctant or scared to do so.

Most young people relax once the assessment begins. With time, they develop a trusting relationship with their health-care professionals. Even in the event that your child carries out this threat and says little, enough useful information can usually be gleaned from the reports and the physical examination to arrive at a working diagnosis.

However, other young people will confess how out of control they feel and how worried they are.

Further questions explore how the eating problems started and progressed, and how the eating problems are affecting their relationships and their ability to function — from their perspective. There will be questions about how they feel about their body image (weight, shape, and size), their friends, and their school life. Questions about their life outside the eating disorder will be asked to explore your child's hopes and dreams.

Nutritional Assessment

During an assessment of the history of your child's food intake, eating attitudes, and behaviors, a dietitian will determine whether your child's diet is adequate in energy, fluids, vitamins, and minerals. Any use of vitamin supplements, caffeine, herbal remedies, and diet products will be evaluated. The dietitian will explore eating patterns, including how many times a day your child usually eats and how much at each meal or snack. Your child's beliefs about food are also examined, especially if your child is a vegetarian, suffers from food allergies, and avoids 'phobic' foods for fear of weight gain or losing control.

During the nutritional assessment, a dietitian will look at any history of binging and purging behaviors. What types and quantities of foods are eaten? What are the frequency and timing of the binge episodes? How does the child feel before and after a binge? What kind of purging method do they use — vomiting, exercise, laxatives, diuretics, weight-control medications?

The dietitian will also ask questions about your family's eating attitudes and behaviors.

Pencil and Paper Questionnaires

In some settings, the assessment team will ask you and your child to complete self-report questionnaires. These questionnaires are often used as additional information to describe and diagnose the eating disorder and other mental health problems.

There are questionnaires that help assess the extent of preoccupation with food, the strength of the drive for thinness, and the extent of the use of various methods to lose weight. They may also assess various personality characteristics frequently associated with eating disorders, such as the level of perfectionism. Other questionnaires specifically focus on the level of depression or anxiety or overall general functioning. The questionnaires are particularly helpful in children and adolescents who are inhibited or anxious during an interview situation.

CASE STUDY Brad

Brad's therapist had been worried about his physical condition and had asked his mother to take him to his pediatrician. He checked his weight and height and plotted them on the pediatric growth curve. It was clear that he had lost weight! The pediatrician suggested a consultation with the Eating Disorder Program at the children's hospital… "just to nip this weight loss in the bud." Brad's family agreed.

They were surprised to learn that there was a waiting list. After waiting 3 months, Brad's family went for their assessment at the Eating Disorder Program. The program was in a children's hospital about an hour away. Brad's family was surprised to discover that there were very few specialized services for kids with eating problems. It seemed like a common problem, at least on television and in the news. They were told to plan on spending the whole day at the hospital. Brad drove with his mother and stepfather in their van, while his father came separately in his own car.

The assessment left everyone's head spinning. First, everyone in the family was seen by a social worker on the team. Then the child psychiatrist met with Brad alone, while the social worker met with the parents. A pediatrician talked with Brad and his parents. This was followed by a physical examination. Brad was then sent to have some blood tests and an EKG to check out his heart rhythm.

The dietitian spoke with Brad and his family about everyone's diet and eating habits.

At the end of this very long day, the team met with Brad and his family. The child psychiatrist reviewed all the information that the team learned that day. They let Brad and his family know that Brad had an eating disorder called Eating Disorder Not Otherwise Specified or ED NOS. The psychiatrist felt that he also had a serious anxiety disorder that was complicating the picture. He needed treatment for both. This would mean a combination of psychotherapy, nutritional counseling, medication, and medical monitoring.

Brad's parents weren't quite sure what all this meant. The team informed Brad and his family that he was very sick and needed close follow-up. The parents didn't hear anything more after that…they were in shock.

continued on page 190

Outcome

After all components of the assessment are complete, the assessment team will meet to review the information, arrive at a working diagnosis, determine the severity of the illness, and develop an initial treatment plan for your child and family. All or several members of the team will then meet with you and your child to discuss the findings.

For some children and adolescents, this may mean immediate hospitalization. For others, it may mean regular outpatient follow-up visits involving a combination of medical monitoring, nutritional support, and individual and family therapy. In still other cases, they may not require intensive treatment and can be followed by their family doctor in their own community.

Use this time to ask any questions you may have. Don't worry about taking up too much time or voicing disagreements to the proposed treatment plan. Everyone has to agree with the plan for it to work.

Parent's Role

The participation of parents in the assessment and treatment of a child with an eating disorder is essential for recovery. You are vital in providing important information about your child and family. You are best equipped to help the assessment team develop a treatment plan that is most likely to be effective. Parents are their child's chief advocates.

You can ensure that your child attends the assessment, insist that all appointments are kept, and make certain that your son or daughter follows through with the recommended treatment. Support them through the difficult times ahead and help them to confront any aspects of the treatment that are uncomfortable or painful.

CHAPTER 12

Choosing a Treatment Strategy

Parenting a child with an eating disorder isn't something that comes naturally to most people. It's likely not something you ever expected to have to do, and the skills involved are not the ones you've needed up to now in your parenting. You're going to need help and good advice. Hardest of all, you are going to have to hand over some aspects of helping your child to other people — not something that comes easily to most parents of a suffering child. To compound this difficulty, parents often receive an onslaught of information from health-care professionals in the early stages of their child's treatment at a time when they are still coming to terms with the diagnosis of an eating disorder and may be overwhelmed by discussions of different treatment options.

Although we have learned a great deal about child and adolescent eating disorders in the last 20 years, there remains a relative lack of scientific information about what treatments are effective. Nevertheless, we have considerable clinical experience in determining what kinds of treatment are best suited to your child and your family. If you or your child should disagree with your treatment team on which treatments are appropriate, be sure to speak up. Other options may be more agreeable and successful.

Treatment Facilities

Assuring your child's medical safety is the first priority of any treatment plan. After an initial medical assessment, your child's doctor or eating disorder team should provide you with a plan for medical care. This may involve immediate inpatient hospitalization, outpatient treatment, day hospitalization (also known as partial hospitalization), or residential treatment.

Hospitalization

If your child is severely malnourished and medically unstable, the necessary and immediate treatment is medical stabilization in hospital, despite whatever objections your child may have.

Moral and Legal Obligations

The adults in a child's life have an obligation to protect that child from making decisions that may have irreversible and negative health consequences. Different parts of the world have different types of legislation that support parents and guardians in this position. There is also a legal obligation for doctors in most jurisdictions to treat patients who are in immediate danger and who cannot make rational decisions about their treatment.

Many experts will tell you that most children, even teenagers, understand this. When told they must be hospitalized, they concede, "So, what you are saying is that I have to stay in hospital and do what you tell me until my heart rate's better, and then I get to choose whether I stay or not?"

Since most young people live at home and are financially dependent on their parents, you will play a major role in the decision-making process about your child's admission to hospital and eligibility for discharge from hospital.

Q: **What if our child refuses to undergo treatment?**

A: How forceful you want to be in trying to persuade your child to accept treatment should be discussed with the eating disorder treatment team. While some children and adolescents will participate in treatment because their parents expect them to, others will not. These deliberations will be shaped by your child's age, developmental stage, the severity and chronicity of her illness, and your beliefs about and approach to parenting. For parents confronting these dilemmas, speaking with other parents who have gone through these trials with their own child may be helpful.

Special Units

Your child will be admitted to a special unit for care: a general pediatric unit, where your child will be with other medically ill children with a variety of diagnoses; a general child and adolescent psychiatric unit, where your child will be with children with other psychiatric disorders; or on a specialized eating disorder unit (either a pediatric eating disorder unit or a combined adolescent and adult eating disorder unit).

The treatment team will comprise some combination of a pediatrician or family doctor, a child psychiatrist, a psychologist, a social worker, child and youth counselors, nurses, a dietitian, an occupational therapist, a physiotherapist, and a teacher. The treatment team will explore factors related to the development of your child's disordered eating. Your son or daughter should also receive an assessment by a doctor regarding their ability to make their own decisions about their treatment.

Sequencing Physical and Psychological Treatments

To start, the focus will be on physical treatments: medical monitoring, refeeding, and weight restoration. A dietitian will educate you and your child about nutritional needs and dispel misconceptions your child may have about food and weight. The staff will support your child at meal times and immediately after meals to avoid purging behaviors, excessive exercise, and food hoarding.

While an inpatient, your child will likely undergo an assessment by a psychiatrist or psychologist who will begin to discuss longer-term psychological treatment options. A psychological assessment will explore the possibility of other psychiatric disorders that may coexist and complicate your child's eating disorder. Your child's motivation to undergo treatment and her ability to benefit from specific psychological interventions will be also assessed.

Some parents of children who are admitted to hospital are surprised if their treatment team does not immediately start intensive psychological treatments. Most treatment teams don't start psychological treatments right away for a number of reasons. Although your son or daughter may have the best intentions in the world, they may not be able to focus or concentrate enough to benefit from intensive psychological treatment because of malnutrition or starvation symptoms. Therefore, the team will initially need to concentrate on medical stabilization through adequate nourishment.

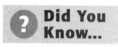

Did You Know...

• The majority of young people admitted to hospital for treatment of eating disorders are malnourished. They may have significant impairments in their ability to think clearly, including trouble with attention and short-term memory.

• Young people with eating disorders may also demonstrate psychological symptoms of starvation, such as food preoccupation, mood swings, and irritability.

Group Programs

If admitted to a specialized eating disorder inpatient unit and when medically fit to do so, your child will likely be expected to participate in group treatments with other young people struggling with eating disorders. Therapists trained to conduct group therapy with expertise in children and adolescent health lead these sessions. The groups may include activity groups, nutrition groups, education groups on eating disorders, and yoga.

Outpatient Programs

When your child is medically stable and ready to return home, the treatment team will plan a comprehensive program for outpatient medical and nutritional monitoring, as well as for some form of psychotherapeutic treatment. The team will refer you to health-care centers and professionals in your community that can provide medical, nutritional, and psychological treatment for your child. In recent years, the range of outpatient options has expanded in some geographic areas.

Day Treatment/Partial Hospitalization Programs

Some areas have day treatment programs (also referred to as partial hospitalization), where your son or daughter eat the majority of their meals in a structured setting during the day and receive psychotherapeutic support from experienced staff. Day treatment is often recommended for children who are unable to succeed in the outpatient programs but do not require the intensive treatment provided on an inpatient unit. These programs offer you and your child the opportunity to learn more about the eating disorder while nutritional and medical needs are closely monitored.

Adolescents rarely accept a day treatment program initially, even if they have had obvious difficulty restoring weight in an inpatient setting and maintaining it on passes home or after discharge as an outpatient. Unless the child is willing to enter a day treatment program, we suggest that parents give their children a second chance as outpatients, explaining that they will be required to enter a day treatment program down the road if progress is not made. Giving your daughter or son the opportunity to show that they can manage to stay out of hospital on their own may be a route worth trying.

Be cautious, however, in giving too many second chances after repeated failures. Adolescents with eating disorders can always come up with plausible reasons why things didn't work this time and why they need another try. Repeated failures after numerous chances might increase your child's risk of prolonging the illness.

CASE STUDY Susan

Susan's parents decided that she needed someone to talk to by herself. Her cousin, who had a "wild" adolescence, was sent to a therapist and did really well. Susan's mother decided to call her sister-in-law to get the name of the therapist. Susan was not interested, but her mother insisted that she go.

The therapist was a nice woman, slightly above average weight. She did something called psychodynamic therapy. Susan's mother liked her right away. Susan was not impressed…all she saw was an overweight person. Susan was worried that the therapist would try and make her fat.

Susan met with the therapist on her own and stubbornly said very little. The therapist said very little as well. Susan told her mother that this was a "complete waste of time and money!"

One month after she started this therapy, the Day Treatment Program called to say they had a place available for Susan. Her parents had put Susan on the waiting list for the Day Treatment Program a few months ago during her hospital admission at the recommendation of the treatment team. This was a back-up plan…just in case. They never expected to need it. Now, they had second thoughts.

Things at home were not great and maybe this could help. They decided to try it. Susan was furious. She refused to go. Susan's father was angry at her refusal. It seemed like she wasn't willing to do anything to get better! Both her parents were adamant that Susan attend the Day Treatment Program, especially if she was planning to live at home. Susan was outraged, but in the end she agreed to go, reluctantly.

This was a huge commitment for Susan and her family. She had to get up early in the morning and would come home rather late in the evening. Susan and her family found the program very helpful and very safe.

But weekends were a challenge. The treatment team saw the weekends as an opportunity for Susan and her family to try out what she had learned during the week. Every weekend, Susan would lose the weight she gained during the week. It was hard not to feel like a failure.

continued on page 203

Residential Programs

If outpatient treatment and day programs do not work for your child and your child requires frequent hospital re-admissions, you may need to look at residential treatment options: residential programs that specialize in eating disorders or residential programs that specialize in general child and adolescent mental health.

Specialized Residential Programs

Residential programs that specialize in treating eating disorders have staff trained not only in adolescent development, but also in the treatment of eating disorders. All the children in these residential programs are suffering from the same type of illness. This can be both a benefit and a drawback. The teens can support each other toward health or illness, depending on the psychological makeup of the group of adolescents in treatment and the program's ability to foster a healthy treatment environment.

General Residential Programs

Adolescents with eating disorders who enter non-specialized residential mental health programs, located close to home, with the hospital providing medical and possibly some part of the psychological treatments, can have success. It tends to be easier to find these types of general residential programs closer to home, which allows parents and siblings to be more closely involved in treatment.

The adolescent with an eating disorder is with other children and adolescents who are less preoccupied with food and weight issues than they are. The other residents' strengths and frailties are more likely to be complementary, rather than identical, to those of adolescents with eating disorders.

Parents tend to be concerned about two issues with these more general residential mental health programs: that their child will be exposed to children with drug, discipline, or other serious mental health problems; and that their child will suffer from the program staff's relative lack of expertise with eating disorders. Both concerns are valid. We recommend strongly that parents assess the residential program for the right fit between their family culture and that of the program before making the decision to enroll their child. We

> **? Did You Know...**
>
> • Residential programs located at a geographic distance may make it difficult for family members to integrate into a treatment plan. This could ultimately interfere with long-term recovery.
>
> • This concern needs to be explored with any residential treatment program you are considering for your child.

would not recommend a program that does not permit a model of care allowing collaboration between the residential staff and the eating disorder experts. The residential staff would take the lead on more general treatment issues relating to the child's mental health, family, and social relationships, while the eating disorder team would make recommendations and possibly provide treatment focused on the eating disorder symptoms.

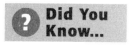

Did You Know...

• There is no single psychological therapy known to be helpful for children, adolescents, and adults with anorexia nervosa.

• Different treatment centers have reported using dance and music therapy, art therapy, guided imagery and relaxation therapies, body image therapies, cognitive-behavioral and interpersonal therapies, psychodynamic psychotherapy, feminist therapy, specific therapies targeting a history of traumatic experiences, and others.

Psychotherapeutic Treatments

In order for children and adolescents to be involved in a psychotherapeutic treatment program, they need to be somewhat motivated or at least able to respond to parent and team recommendations. You need to spend time understanding what kinds of treatment your child is both suited for and willing to tolerate. There is nothing more irritating to adolescents — particularly with an eating disorder that they aren't sure they want to give up — to be told by an adult, whom they do not necessarily know or trust, and without being consulted first, that they need a time-consuming and demanding psychological treatment.

Psychotherapeutic treatment will likely consist of your child talking to a therapist or talking with a group therapist and other children suffering from an eating disorder about psychological experiences related to the illness. Family therapy may also be recommended, particularly where the child or adolescent's motivation is in question.

A good psychological assessment will look at your child's fit with different types of therapy. A highly articulate adolescent may be the perfect candidate for a talking therapy; alternatively, it may be important for adolescents to challenge themselves to explore more body-focused or non-verbal therapies if they have a tendency to neglect these aspects of their experience.

Let's look in depth at some of the most successful psychological therapies — family therapy, cognitive-behavior therapy, interpersonal therapy, and motivation enhancement therapy.

You Can Help...

We hesitate to add to your burdens, but we strongly encourage you to give family psychoeducation and family therapy a chance. These are the best ways to support your family and your child with an eating disorder through a long and difficult illness — and the best way to support the family as a whole through the inevitable stress that accompanies the illness.

Family Therapy

The only psychotherapeutic treatments that have been validated for younger adolescents under the age of 18 are parent counseling and family therapy. Subsequent research studies have demonstrated that whether the family therapy focuses on education about eating disorders — called family psychoeducation — or uses discussion of family relationships and roles, it can be equally effective. It is rare for children or adolescents with eating disorders, and rarer still for their siblings, to express much enthusiasm for family therapy. Faced with an ill child whom they are desperately trying to enlist in treatment, parents often find it difficult to insist on attendance. Indeed parents' own challenges with juggling work and other family commitments may result in family therapy falling to the bottom of their list of preferred treatments.

Q: What if my daughter refuses to attend family therapy sessions?

A: If your child is young or an early adolescent, then it is entirely appropriate for you to insist, in the same way that you would insist she take an antibiotic prescribed by her doctor. For an older adolescent, you may decide to give her the chance to do it her way, but with clear expectations that you will re-evaluate after a specific amount of time. For example, "Fine, we are going to try it your way. No family therapy if you can continue to restore your weight out of hospital...but if 2 months from now you are still struggling, we're going to do it our way."

While you are waiting to see how things play out in the latter scenario, we recommend that you become involved in parent counseling or a parent support group — if either is provided in your treatment center — where you can share experiences with and seek advice from other parents of children with eating disorders.

Some eating disorder programs may suggest that you start family therapy whether you child attends or not. Often in this situation, part of the work is focused on how to get your daughter or son to participate in the family therapy.

PSYCHOLOGICAL TREATMENT OPTIONS

Let's start with a child or adolescent who is ready for outpatient treatment, either because they have successfully completed an inpatient admission or because they are medically well enough to remain out of hospital and appear sufficiently motivated to recover that you and the treatment team don't need to consider more intensive treatment at this time. What are your options?

Psychotherapy

Aims to help an individual, family, or a group of adolescents to become aware of links between their thoughts and feelings and their symptoms. Includes family therapy, cognitive-behavior therapy, and interpersonal therapy.

Family Psychoeducation

Involves teaching parents and their child with an eating disorder about eating disorders, how to treat them, and how to recognize signs of relapse. This therapy also teaches coping strategies and problem-solving skills to help deal more effectively with the child and the eating disorder.

Family Therapy

Involves the child with the eating disorder, the parents, and a therapist. Brothers and sisters, as well as other relatives, may also be included. This therapy emphasizes an understanding of the roles and relationships of each member of the family system. The goal of family therapy is to work on making changes in how your family functions as a unit, so that you and your child can better fight the eating disorder or any other difficulties that may arise. It also can help with treatment planning and provide a way to offer the family support and understanding in a time of crisis. Family therapy is the only psychotherapeutic treatment that has been validated for adolescents under the age of 18.

Cognitive-Behavior Therapy (CBT)

Encourages patients to look at how the way they think influences their feelings and behavior, possibly in self-destructive, negative, or simply unhelpful ways. CBT is the most widely used individual treatment for eating disorders. It has been shown to be effective in young adults with bulimia nervosa.

Interpersonal Therapy (IPT)

Focuses on patients' relationships with the important people in their lives, specifically more difficult relationships and how they may affect eating disorder symptoms. IPT has been show to be effective in adults with eating disorders.

Motivation Enhancement Therapy (MET)

Accepts patients' expressed readiness for change and works with them to identify areas of their life that might improve if they took on the eating disorder more forcefully. More suited for older adolescents.

Art and Play Therapy

Allows younger children to experiment with different art forms and to play with a variety of toys that might reflect their feelings and reveal issues affecting their lives.

Relaxation Therapies

Aim to improve the patient's ability to relax both physically and mentally. These therapies include deep breathing, stretching, muscle relaxation, and guided imagery.

Guided Imagery

Helps patients to visualize in their imagination, using all their senses, images of safety or comfort that they can then use to help them relax and to manage difficult thoughts and feelings without resorting to self-destructive behaviors. An example might be a young woman who is feeling stressed. Instead of reacting to the stress by binging, she imagines a place in her mind where she feels safe and in control. This therapy has shown some benefit to patients with bulimia nervosa.

Body Image Therapy

Helps patients to experience their bodies in new, less critical ways — some body-focused, some relaxation strategies, some cognitive-behavioral techniques, and others.

Psychodynamic Psychotherapy

Relates the patient's current experience to past experiences and relationships in an attempt to clarify deeper or buried motivations for current behaviors.

Feminist Therapy

Explores the patient's symptoms in the context of gender roles and power relationships between men and women in society. Used extensively in the treatment of eating disorders.

Mindfulness Therapy

Employs techniques used in some Eastern religions, such as detachment from feelings, observing oneself, meditation, and focusing on the present, to assist patients in relaxing and becoming more aware of how and when symptoms emerge in their lives. Some initial research demonstrates this may be useful for patients with bulimic and binge-eating symptoms.

Meditation

Using deep breathing and focusing of one's mind to instill relaxation.

Individual and Group Psychotherapies

In addition to family therapy, health-care professionals use several individual and group therapies that have been demonstrated to be helpful in other childhood mental illnesses, such as depression and anxiety disorders, and to work for adults with eating disorders. We are forced to rely on these sources because of the dearth of specific scientific information on psychological treatments for children and teenagers with eating disorders.

Many clinicians believe that adolescents with eating disorders benefit from group therapy because it allows them to grapple with social issues they have with peers in a safer setting. Group therapy also allows young people to experience the relief of finding out that other teenagers struggle with similar issues.

There are adolescents, who for reasons related to shyness or shame, insist on individual therapy. It's not worth arguing over. If your daughter or son is one of these adolescents, be pleased they are accepting treatment and come back later to the group therapy idea if you think it's important. During individual treatments, your child's reluctance to join a group may be explored.

Art and Play Therapy

For young children, family therapy is almost always the treatment of choice, but may be supplemented by art or play therapy. Both therapies have been used extensively with children for a variety of psychological disorders. Art therapists introduce your child to a variety of art forms — painting, collage, and clay sculpting, to name a few — and encourage the child to use them during the treatment session. The therapist may talk with your son or daughter about how the artwork seems to reflect issues and feelings in their lives. The play therapist introduces the child to a number of different toys and games, and will also, if appropriate, link the child's play with life outside the treatment session.

Cognitive-Behavior Therapy

Cognitive-behavior therapy (CBT) is starting to be used for adolescents with a variety of psychiatric disorders, such as depression and anxiety, as well as for adolescents with eating disorders.

CBT encourages patients to look at how their way of thinking influences their feelings and behavior, possibly in

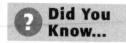
Did You Know...

• Some parents worry that their child will pick up more eating disordered behaviors and attitudes in a group setting.

• Although this is a risk, young people with eating disorders are likely to have discovered everything there is to know about 'pro' weight-loss beliefs and strategies from numerous sources available to them. This information is widely available in the books and magazines they read, on the Internet sites they surf, and from their groups of friends...long before they seek treatment.

self-destructive, negative, or simply unhelpful ways. For example, a 'perfectionist' adolescent will tend to measure herself against impossibly high standards, and therefore feel doomed to failure and disappointment. A 'black and white thinker' may look at issues only in terms of right or wrong, or success and failure, again causing her to judge herself and others excessively harshly.

Identifying some of these so-called 'cognitive distortions' — in which facts and experiences are reshaped to fit to a person's self-image or world view — can improve someone's self-assessment and perspective on relationships. These changes can, in turn, encourage patients to feel more confident and optimistic about their ability to overcome illness-related symptoms.

During the behavior aspect of the therapy, the therapist encourages patients to make shifts to new behaviors based on these changes in their thinking. An example might be to encourage a perfectionist adolescent to hand in a piece of homework she feels is imperfect, then to explore with her how that experience feels.

CBT benefits teenagers who are already motivated to challenge their beliefs about themselves and their eating behaviors. It usually involves homework between sessions.

CBT can be delivered through individual therapy (one-on-one treatment) and group therapy (with a group of other people suffering from an eating disorder).

Interpersonal Therapy

Interpersonal therapy (IPT) focuses on patients' relationships with the important people in their lives and how they may affect their eating disorder symptoms. For children or adolescents to benefit from IPT, they need to be willing to talk about these relationships. Adolescent girls who tend to place a high value on relationships seem to do well with IPT; some boys may find it harder to use this type of therapy because of their tendency to minimize the importance of their relationships early on in therapy.

IPT therapy can be quite effective, for example, in adolescents with bulimia nervosa who are in constant conflict with their parents. Every conversation they have with their parents ends up in a fight, leaving them feeling misunderstood, frustrated, and bad about themselves. To cope with this feeling, they binge and purge. The therapist intercedes to examine this parent-child relationship and to assist them in

? Did You Know...

● Research on adults with eating disorders has demonstrated that both cognitive-behavior therapy (CBT) and interpersonal therapy (IPT) can be helpful for older adolescents and adults struggling with bulimia nervosa and binge eating disorder.

improving their verbal and non-verbal communication. As the conflict subsides and the relationship with the parents improves, they have less need to cope by binging and purging. Although the focus of the therapy is specific, adolescents will learn new coping and relationship skills that they can use throughout their lives.

Like CBT, IPT can be delivered through individual therapy (one-on-one treatment) and group therapy (with a group of other people suffering from an eating disorder).

Motivation Enhancement Therapy

An adolescent who has no interest in recovery should not necessarily be excluded from therapy. Motivation enhancement therapy (MET), based on work with patients suffering from addictions, may be helpful for these patients. While accepting this expressed lack of interest in changing, therapists assist young people in identifying areas of their lives that might improve if they took on their eating disorder more forcefully.

MET, without any other forms of therapy, is more suited for older adolescents. With younger children, it is developmentally essential for parents to set out clear expectations and not to accept a "no" to treatment. However, with a 17-year-old daughter who has not benefited from other treatments, it may be developmentally appropriate for you to allow her the opportunity to explore with a therapist her reluctance to work toward recovery.

Therapies for Coexisting Psychological Problems

If a child or adolescent with an eating disorder suffers from coexisting psychological difficulties — the most common being anxiety and depression — the treatment team will likely recommend specific therapies shown to be effective in treating these disorders. Unless these other problems are addressed, the child is unlikely to achieve recovery.

An example of a therapy recommended for a coexisting problem would be the use of cognitive-behavior therapy (CBT) to treat obsessive-compulsive disorder. CBT is a therapy that has proven in research studies to be effective for children and adolescents with this problem and others. Another example may be the use of medication to treat a depression.

CASE STUDY Martha

Martha's treatment team recommended cognitive behavioral therapy, explaining to her and her parents that it can work well for young adults struggling with bulimia nervosa.

For Martha, the good news was that there were only 16 sessions that she was required to attend. She went to her first appointment, reluctantly, but liked the therapist right away. She was less sure about the treatment. The therapist was clear that if this treatment was going to work, Martha would have to make a serious commitment to the process. This would take hard work and there would be homework. This sounded like school...and Martha already felt like she had enough of that!

She told her parents that she had doubts about committing to this program, but her parents told her it was time for her to take responsibility for herself. It was time Martha grew up!

Martha decided to give it a shot. She went to the sessions regularly. Most of the time she got her homework done. There were a lot of charts to fill out about her eating, binging, and purging, lots of questions about her thoughts and feelings. Slowly, the charts helped her understand her behavior patterns. She began to see how her automatic thinking patterns affected her feelings and her behaviors. She learned to change some of her thinking.

Remarkably, things in her life started to improve. Before she knew it, the 16 sessions were over. Martha was sad to say goodbye to her therapist. Now everyone was watching to see what she could do on her own.

continued on page 243

Medications

Some children and adolescents with eating disorders may also benefit from medication. However, these medications need to be administered with caution to insure their effectiveness and safety.

Most discussions of psychiatric medications tend to make parents and children anxious, especially following recent reports that certain antidepressant medications prescribed for children and adolescents may increase the risk for self-harm impulses and suicidal thoughts. A number of governments have restricted and even banned the use of these medications in children and adolescents until these studies can be thoroughly reviewed.

We are hopeful that with further research, a wider range of successful and safe psychopharmacological treatments for children and adolescents with eating disorders will become available. However, at this time, the selective serotonin reuptake inhibitors and atypical antipsychotic medications are the only ones that have demonstrated anything approaching a consistently helpful effect.

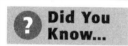

? Did You Know...

• At this stage in medical research, there is no clear-cut scientific information that any psychiatric medication is helpful to adolescents with anorexia nervosa, especially when the adolescent remains at a low weight.

Selective Serotonin Reuptake Inhibitors

There is some indication that selective serotonin reuptake inhibitors (SSRIs), used to treat depression and anxiety, may be helpful in preventing relapse in older adolescents and adults with eating disorders who have already restored their weight to a healthy level.

SSRIs, specifically fluoxetine, have been shown to be helpful in higher doses than are usually used for depression or anxiety, for adults with bulimia nervosa and binge eating disorders. In addition, there is some early evidence that SSRIs, an appetite suppressant called sibutramine, and topiramate (currently used for patients with seizures, migraine headaches, and mood disorders) may be helpful for adult patients with binge eating disorders.

However, SSRIs are among the medications under review by a number of government drug regulatory agencies. They should only be considered for a trial of medication when a child or adolescent with an eating disorder has consistently demonstrated difficulty maintaining the progress achieved after hospitalization; when other therapies have not proven effective; or when the patient has a coexisting psychiatric illness known to respond to these medications.

Atypical Neuroleptic Medications

There are some reports that other medications currently used to treat a variety of childhood psychiatric and behavioral disorders and originally developed for treatment of psychotic disorders may help children and adolescents with eating disorders to gain weight and to reduce their anxiety and obsessional thinking. These medications are known as atypical neuroleptic medications. The most commonly used of these medications include risperidone, olanzapine, and quetiapine.

Since these medications have significant side effects, pediatric psychiatrists consider their use primarily in children and adolescents who have been unsuccessful in maintaining any semblance of normal life outside hospital, who are requiring serial hospitalizations because of the severity of their eating disorder, or who suffer from a coexisting psychiatric illness where these medications are a necessary treatment.

Medication Pros and Cons

You are right to be cautious about treating your child's eating disorder with medication. The majority of research on the use of psychiatric medications in the treatment of eating disorders has been obtained from studies done in adults; we have limited information on their use in children and adolescents. SSRIs may induce thoughts of self-harm and suicide in a small number of children to whom they are prescribed. SSRIs and atypical neuroleptics have side effects that need to be considered before a trial of the medication can be recommended. Furthermore, these side effects need to be carefully monitored if this treatment modality is used.

Be assured that doctors are familiar with appropriate doses and side effects. If they prescribe these medications for your child, they will monitor your child for the emergence of common and serious side effects by asking questions, doing physical examinations, and ordering laboratory tests. These procedures will all be helpful in identifying and treating any side effects that do occur.

Your doctor should inform you and your child about the benefits and risks of the medications being recommended. You should monitor your child for any side effects from the medication and report them to your doctor.

Having acknowledged all of these reasons to be cautious, it is important for us to emphasize that eating disorders are difficult to treat and life-threatening. Many patients who take psychiatric medications do not experience side-effects and the most serious side effects are rare.

Adding medication to the treatment plan when your child is struggling, despite everyone's best efforts, may improve the course of this persistent illness or prevent the illness from becoming so serious that it will negatively affect the remainder of your child's life or even threaten your child's very life.

WHAT IF I DISAGREE WITH THE TREATMENT RECOMMENDATIONS?

If you disagree with the treatments recommended by the treatment team and your child is medically stable, you have a number of options:

1. Sometimes disagreements are based on miscommunication or misunderstandings that can be resolved by further meetings and discussion with your child's treatment team. Ask the team to explain its rationale for these recommendations again.

2. If you continue to disagree, you can ask for another opinion from other health-care professionals with expertise in eating disorders not currently involved with your child's treatment team.

3. If that second opinion is not satisfactory to you, you can request a transfer of care to a different health-care facility or health-care team. You will likely want to explore the availability of the alternatives in your community before making such a decision. Consider carefully your child's relationship with the current treatment team and whether she has an attachment to certain people that will be disrupted by a change. Good relationships between health-care professionals and your child are essential for recovery. These relationships may not be easy to replace elsewhere.

You may never feel that you have enough information to feel entirely confident in your decision about using medications, but now you will know that you have made it to the best of your ability.

Look After Yourself

Busy hospital wards and doctors' offices are not conducive to calm reflection. Consider different treatment options at a pace and a time of your choosing. Take the time to think about what you've read, to discuss it with your co-parent, your friends, other health-care professionals, or your child, as you see fit. Talk to your child's treatment team about what you've read and ask them what they see as likely to be helpful for your child.

Be sure to look after yourself and to seek the support you need to make these decisions well. Most children with eating disorders will get better but it may take 5 years or longer. The road to recovery from an eating disorder is long and arduous for your child and your family; it demands both stamina and persistence.

With education and support you will know which treatment decisions are life and death ones and how to respond to those appropriately. For the others, there is rarely one answer that's right or wrong; more often, finding the right treatments involves trying different approaches and judging when to move on to something else. Knowing this will help you keep a big picture perspective rather than getting trapped by the belief that a single treatment is the only hope for recovery.

CHAPTER 13

Learning to Eat Again

Eating well again and maintaining a healthy weight are fundamental to any treatment program for children and adolescents with eating disorders. Combine good nutrition with moderate physical activity and a positive self-image and the stage is set for recovery.

None of this is easy, however. Young people with eating disorders develop unusual ideas about what good nutrition means, and many individuals find maintaining a healthy weight challenging, especially if they are still restricting their food intake, binging, or purging. Physical activity may become excessive or unhealthy as they try to maintain weight loss. Any gain in weight, no matter how healthy, can reinforce any negative attitudes they may have about their physical appearance.

So, how do we teach these children and adolescents to eat well again? Better yet, how do we help them to learn this for themselves? To eat a nutritionally well-balanced diet, their relationship with food needs to change. For them to set their sights on a healthy weight, they also need to revise the body image the eating disorder has created in their mind. And for them to exercise in a healthy way, they need to understand the need for moderation and find the fun again in their physical activities.

Helping your child to work through these challenges of learning to eat normally, maintaining a healthy weight, and enjoying healthy activity is vital for recovery.

What Is Good Nutrition?

If your child has an eating disorder, it is sometimes helpful, especially early on, to think of food as your child's medicine. Your child may not want to eat the food, but it is necessary in order to move toward recovery.

Meal Plans

In the initial stages of treatment, your daughter or son will often need to eat mechanically — that is, they will have to eat meals with set amounts of food at specific times of day, whether they feel hungry or not.

Many times, when children or adolescents with eating disorders start following a meal plan after a long period of starvation or chaotic eating, they may feel too full or even experience bloating or cramps after eating only small amounts because the digestion system has slowed down due to lack of activity. Often they interpret these physical symptoms as a reason to eat less when, in fact, the only cure for these symptoms is to keep eating according to their structured meal times and amounts. Consistent eating helps the digestive system be more active, working it into shape like other muscles in the body.

Your child's meal plan should include a variety of foods that provide all the nutrients required for normal development and good health. Nutrients are chemical substances, found in food, that nourish the body and help keep it in good working order.

Over time, your daughter or son will use their meal plan to increase their intake if required, to diversify the foods they are willing to eat, and to eat more regularly. The meal plan should also help your child to feel more normal patterns of hunger and fullness.

Your child's ultimate goal is to learn how to eat intuitively three non-dieting meals and two to three snacks a day to meet their energy needs. It does take a lot of hard work in the beginning, but, in time, it should become a normal part of their day.

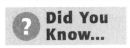

Did You Know...

● Most children and adolescents with eating disorders have lost the ability to eat instinctively or intuitively. They cannot rely on their hunger or fullness sensations to guide their eating.

● They may no longer be aware of these sensations or they may feel compelled to ignore these sensations due to the pressure of the eating disorder.

VALUE OF MEAL PLANS

Learning to eat mechanically involves the use of a structured meal plan. A meal plan is a useful guide to help restore normal eating patterns.

● Provides structure and safety

● Promotes meal regularity

● Focuses on meeting your child's energy needs

● Contains portions that reflect those of normal eaters

● Provides all of the nutrients necessary for growth, activity, and psychological well-being

● Promotes eating normally and eating a variety of different foods

● Helps your child resist the temptation to count calories and grams of fat

● With time and support, allows eating to become natural and intuitive instead of mechanical

HELP FOR STRUCTURING A MEAL PLAN

Placing appropriate limits and expectations on your child's eating behaviors from the beginning is crucial. Create a safe environment for eating. This is done with a structured meal plan.

- Create and maintain a non-dieting environment at home. The home should be a diet-free zone, where different body shapes and sizes are accepted.

- Become aware of your own personal attitudes and issues about food and weight. Become a model of healthy eating attitudes and behaviors.

- Work together to support your child.

- Try to make meals as supportive as possible by finding out what is helpful or not helpful for your son or daughter.

- Mealtimes can be stressful, so avoid topics that may cause anxiety.

- Be aware of how casual comments about eating may be interpreted. Avoid comments like this, "Wow, I haven't seen you eat a piece of cake in years!"

- Consider planning meals and snacks 2 to 3 days in advance with your child to provide structure. This will help to decrease anxiety. Once this plan has been established, changes should be kept to a minimum. This will encourage your child to take responsibility for their choices and start to become more flexible with their eating.

- At school, it may be helpful to arrange for someone to sit with your daughter or son and support them during meal and snack times.

- Consistently prepare and serve nutritionally balanced meals to the entire family.

- Sit down with the family for meals as often as you can. Mealtime is a wonderful place to reconnect with your family members and talk about things other than weight and food.

- Teach your child to become accepting of all kinds of people.

- Teach your children to become accepting of themselves and their special qualities.

- Encourage your son or daughter to believe in their strengths.

Food Guides

A meal plan commonly includes three meals and two to three snacks that offer all the nutrients children and adolescents require for good health. Meal plans are based on eating a well-balanced diet from the main food groups described in the *Food Guide Pyramid: A Guide to Daily Food Choices*, issued by the United States Department of Agriculture, or *Canada's Food Guide to Healthy Eating*, issued by Health Canada.

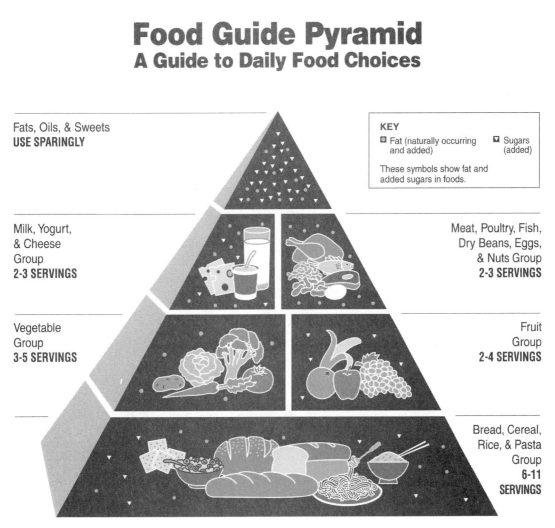

Food Guide Pyramid
A Guide to Daily Food Choices

Fats, Oils, & Sweets
USE SPARINGLY

KEY
▢ Fat (naturally occurring and added)   ▼ Sugars (added)

These symbols show fat and added sugars in foods.

Milk, Yogurt, & Cheese Group
2-3 SERVINGS

Meat, Poultry, Fish, Dry Beans, Eggs, & Nuts Group
2-3 SERVINGS

Vegetable Group
3-5 SERVINGS

Fruit Group
2-4 SERVINGS

Bread, Cereal, Rice, & Pasta Group
6-11 SERVINGS

Source: U.S. Department of Agriculture/U.S. Department of Health and Human Services

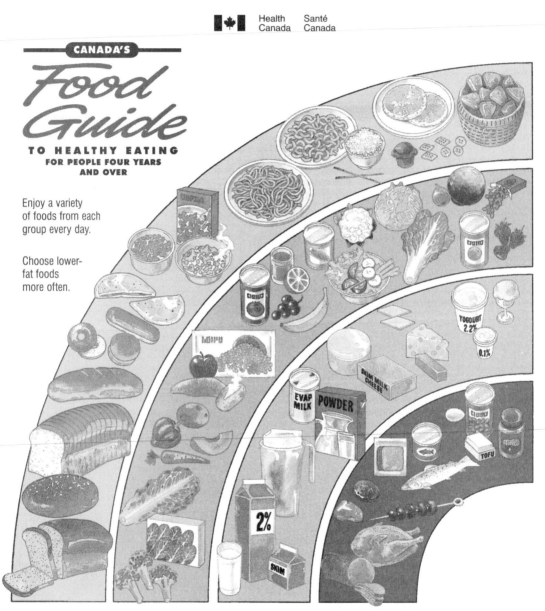

Health   Santé
Canada   Canada

CANADA'S
Food Guide
TO HEALTHY EATING
FOR PEOPLE FOUR YEARS
AND OVER

Enjoy a variety
of foods from each
group every day.

Choose lower-
fat foods
more often.

Grain Products
Choose whole grain
and enriched
products more often.

Vegetables and Fruit
Choose dark green and
orange vegetables and
orange fruit more often.

Milk Products
Choose lower-fat milk
products more often.

Meat and Alternatives
Choose leaner meats,
poultry and fish, as well
as dried peas, beans
and lentils more often.

Canada

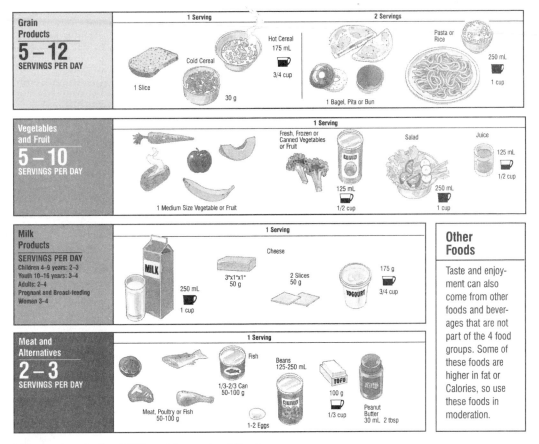

| Grain Products **5 – 12** SERVINGS PER DAY | 1 Serving: 1 Slice, Cold Cereal 30 g, Hot Cereal 175 mL 3/4 cup | 2 Servings: 1 Bagel, Pita or Bun, Pasta or Rice 250 mL 1 cup |

Vegetables and Fruit **5 – 10** SERVINGS PER DAY — 1 Serving: 1 Medium Size Vegetable or Fruit; Fresh, Frozen or Canned Vegetables or Fruit 125 mL 1/2 cup; Salad 250 mL 1 cup; Juice 125 mL 1/2 cup

Milk Products — SERVINGS PER DAY — Children 4–9 years: 2–3; Youth 10–16 years: 3–4; Adults: 2–4; Pregnant and Breast-feeding Women 3–4 — 1 Serving: MILK 250 mL 1 cup; Cheese 3"x1"x1" 50 g, 2 Slices 50 g; 175 g YOGOURT 3/4 cup

Meat and Alternatives **2 – 3** SERVINGS PER DAY — 1 Serving: Meat, Poultry or Fish 50-100 g; Fish 1/3-2/3 Can 50-100 g; 1-2 Eggs; Beans 125-250 mL; TOFU 100 g; Peanut Butter 30 mL 2 tbsp 1/3 cup

Other Foods

Taste and enjoyment can also come from other foods and beverages that are not part of the 4 food groups. Some of these foods are higher in fat or Calories, so use these foods in moderation.

Different People Need Different Amounts of Food

The amount of food you need every day from the 4 food groups and other foods depends on your age, body size, activity level, whether you are male or female and if you are pregnant or breast-feeding. That's why the Food Guide gives a lower and higher number of servings for each food group. For example, young children can choose the lower number of servings, while male teenagers can go to the higher number. Most other people can choose servings somewhere in between.

Consult *Canada's Physical Activity Guide to Healthy Active Living* to help you build physical activity into your daily life.

Enjoy eating well, being active and feeling good about yourself. That's VITALIT ®.

© Minister of Public Works and Government Services Canada, 1997
Cat. No. H39-252/1992E   ISBN 0-662-19648-1

Nutrients

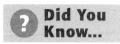
Carbohydrates

Carbohydrates are the body's main source of energy. Carbohydrates are used to make fuel for cells in muscles, the brain, and the nervous system. They are classified into two groups: simple (sugars) and complex (starches) carbohydrates. A healthy diet should include both simple and complex carbohydrates. Some of the body's tissues, like the brain and muscles, can *only* use carbohydrates to function.

Simple carbohydrate foods provide an instant source of energy because they are digested and absorbed rapidly. They include milk products, fruit, table sugar, honey, and jam.

Complex carbohydrates take longer to digest, so they can help us to feel full for a longer period of time. They include breads, cereals, pasta, rice, potatoes, and beans.

Fiber is also considered a carbohydrate, although it is not an energy source because the body does not digest it. Fiber helps move solid wastes through the digestive tract. Fiber helps with constipation and aids in digestion. Fiber can be found in whole grain products, oats, beans, fruits, and vegetables.

Fat

Despite what we hear in the media, our bodies need fat to work. Children need to eat fat to grow properly and for normal brain development. Fat provides energy and essential fatty acids that our body cannot produce. It helps to deliver and absorb the fat-soluble vitamins A, D, E, and K. Fat also provides the construction material for cells and hormones. In addition, fat helps satisfy hunger by making us feel full after eating and it also makes food taste better. Examples of fat include butter, margarine, oils, sour cream, and mayonnaise.

Fats that people eat are a combination of two different types: saturated fat and unsaturated fat. Saturated fats are found mostly in animal foods (fatty meats, whole milk products, egg yolk, butter, and lard) and tropical oils (palm and coconut oils). Unsaturated fats are found mostly in nuts and nut butters, seeds, vegetable and olive oils, and avocados.

Unsaturated fat can be monounsaturated or polyunsaturated. Monounsaturated fat is found mostly in canola, peanut and olive oils, nuts, seeds, and avocados. Polyunsaturated fat is found mostly in nuts and seeds, as well as in corn, safflower, and sunflower oils. Omega-3 fats are a type of polyunsaturated fat that is required by the body. It is found in some fish and fish oils, flaxseed, canola and soybean oils, and omega-3 enriched eggs.

Many foods contain both types of fat (saturated and unsaturated). A healthy diet should include all kinds of fat in moderation, though, overall, you should aim for your child to have more unsaturated fat (mono and poly) than saturated and trans fat in their diet. Trans fatty acids should also be avoided. They occur naturally in small amounts in some animal foods, but are also created when liquid vegetable oils are turned into partially solid fat by a method called partial hydrogenation. Food companies often use this method of hydrogenation to help preserve foods. Foods made with partially hydrogenated oil or shortening, including crackers, chips, cookies, and french fries, may contain trans fats.

> **? Did You Know...**
>
> • Bones, organs, muscles, hair, nails, teeth, and skin are all made up of protein.

Protein

Protein is essential for life, providing the body with the building materials for growth and repair of body tissues. Proteins are involved in the formation of antibodies (which help fight illness and disease) and hormones. Proteins also provide energy when carbohydrates and fat are in short supply. However, if they're used for energy, they can't be used to maintain body tissue.

Ensuring appropriate protein intake during adolescence is important. Protein is found in such foods as meats, fish, milk products, eggs, peanut butter, beans (including soy products), seeds, and nuts.

Q: My daughter has been trying to normalize her eating. I'm unsure about planning her meals and snacks. What should I include in her meals and snacks and how much should she be eating?

A: Review the *Food Guide Pyramid: A Guide to Daily Food Choices*, issued by the United States Department of Agriculture, or *Canada's Food Guide to Healthy Eating*, issued by Health Canada.

A normal meal should include portions from the following food groups. If your child has a meal plan, it can be used to learn what appropriate portion sizes look like. You can also base the size of portions on what other normal eaters are eating. Check off each group as you prepare a meal.

☐ Protein   ☐ Carbohydrates
☐ Fat   ☐ Fruit or vegetable or both
☐ Milk product   ☐ Dessert

A normal snack usually includes 2 to 3 of these groups (for example: 1 piece of fruit + 1 muffin or 1 peanut butter sandwich + 1 cup of milk).

Water

Water is an important nutrient that is often overlooked. Approximately two-thirds of body weight is water. Water transports nutrients and waste products in the body, aids in digestion, and helps regulate body temperature and blood pressure. Six to 10 cups of non-caffeinated, non-alcoholic fluids are required daily to maintain proper fluid balance. These fluids include water, juice, milk, and other non-caffeinated drinks.

Vitamins and Minerals

Vitamins and minerals do not provide energy but help the body use the energy from carbohydrates, fat, and protein. In addition, vitamins and minerals act as spark plugs, setting off many other chemical reactions in the body that help it to function normally.

Each vitamin and mineral has a unique role, and therefore the body requires all of them in certain amounts. A varied diet or meal plan should provide all the vitamins and minerals required. However, there are some minerals of particular concern for adolescents.

Calcium

Calcium is a mineral that helps build strong bones and healthy teeth. It also helps with blood clotting and proper functioning of the nerves, muscles, and heart. Calcium-rich foods include milk, yogurt, cheese, ice cream, tofu processed with calcium, and calcium-fortified juices.

Many research studies report that healthy teens, let alone teens with eating disorders, do not consume adequate amounts of calcium. Inadequate calcium intake may be putting their bones at risk for long-term complications, such as osteoporosis, a condition where the bones weaken and become brittle, breaking more easily.

Calcium doesn't work alone. It works with other nutrients, including vitamin D and phosphorus. Phosphorus helps to form and to maintain strong bones and teeth. Vitamin D helps the body use calcium and phosphorus, which makes bones and teeth stronger. Ensuring children and teenagers get adequate calcium and vitamin D in their diets is vital.

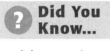

Did You Know...

• Adolescence is a critical time for bone growth and development. Almost half of an adult's bone mass is formed during the teen years.

• Adolescents need extra calcium to accumulate an optimal amount of bone. They require the equivalent of 4 cups of milk per day to meet their calcium requirements.

Iron

Iron is a mineral we all need to keep our bodies functioning at their best. Teenagers have increased needs for iron during puberty due to rapid growth, and, for females, due to the iron losses from menstruation.

Iron works by helping to form hemoglobin, which is an important part of red blood cells. Hemoglobin carries oxygen to all parts of the body. Without enough iron, the body cells get less oxygen. This can cause someone to look pale and feel tired, weak and irritable.

Iron can be found in animal and plant products. Iron from meat, poultry, and fish is better absorbed by the body than the iron from plant sources, such as beans, lentils, spinach, nuts, and seeds. However, absorption of iron from plants can be improved by eating fruit or drinking juice that contains vitamin C with the iron-rich food.

What About Vegetarian Diets?

Vegetarian diets are becoming more popular, but raise concerns for parents of children and adolescents with eating disorders. A well-planned vegetarian diet can supply the body with enough energy and nutrients, as long as foods are chosen carefully. Poorly planned vegetarian diets may be lacking in energy, protein, iron, calcium, vitamin D, vitamin B12, and zinc because certain foods or food groups are omitted from the diet.

There are many reasons young people choose to become a vegetarian: concern over animal rights, concern over the environment, religious beliefs, family beliefs, lifestyle factors, and health issues are among the most common. Sometimes teenagers choose vegetarianism as an excuse to diet, to lose weight, or to take control of their life in the area of food. If that is the case, you may have a child who may be developing an eating disorder.

If your child claims to be a vegetarian, avoids food groups without getting enough nutrients from other foods, and is not able to maintain a healthy weight, then this may be a symptom of an eating disorder. Teenagers with an eating disorder may associate vegetarianism with a low-fat and low-energy diet; therefore use vegetarianism as a way of controlling their food intake and their weight.

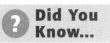

Did You Know...

• Many teens, especially girls, don't get enough iron due to poor food choices or restricting food intake to lose weight.

• Adolescents who don't eat meat may also find it difficult to get enough iron in their diets.

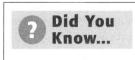

Did You Know...

There are different types of vegetarian diets.

• **Vegan** diets avoid all foods of animal origin, including eggs, dairy products, honey, and gelatin.

• **Lacto-ovo Vegetarian** diets avoid all animal flesh, but include eggs and dairy products.

• **Semi-vegetarian** diets generally avoid red meat, but include fish, poultry, eggs, and dairy products.

If your daughter or son chooses to become a vegetarian, try to understand the reasons why they have made this choice. The most important thing you can do is to educate yourself and make sure that the foods that are omitted are substituted with nutritionally adequate replacements. A dietitian can help to ensure that your child's vegetarian diet is complete.

CASE STUDY Brad

After his initial eating disorder assessment, Brad and his parents were given a meal plan — very structured with three meals and three snacks a day, with suggestions for what constituted a reasonable meal and snack. Brad and his parents were perplexed…exactly how was this going to work? Nobody ate like this. It wasn't normal. The dietitian explained that this was called "mechanical eating" and was the first step to eating normally.

A week later, Brad and his family returned to the clinic. Brad's weight hadn't changed. His mother was concerned because Brad had lots of food rules about what he called "safe" foods and "scary" foods. There were very few foods on the list that he agreed to eat! In fact, he ended up eating the same thing, at the same time every day. The dietitian reassured the parents that this was not unusual at this stage of the eating disorder.

Over the next few weeks, the team encouraged Brad and his parents to take "baby steps." They would slowly work on helping him break his food rules and try new foods. Small rewards would be put in place when he did what was expected and logical consequences would result when he was unable to follow through. The team worked with Brad and his parents to come up with the rewards and consequences.

But before they could institute the plan for breaking the food rules, the team asked to meet with the parents. They had some concerns. Brad was not gaining weight. Some weeks he would be up, some weeks he would be down. What was going on? Then they figured it out.

His mother, who was pregnant, woke up in the middle of the night to go to the bathroom. She caught Brad exercising frantically in his room. It turned out that Brad wasn't afraid of gaining weight, but he was exercising to make sure that all his weight gain was muscle and not fat. He wanted to have a 'six-pack' physique.

continued on page 255

Snack Foods and Desserts

Snack foods and desserts should also be included in your child's meal plan. Examples of snack foods and desserts include cookies, brownies, ice cream, chips, chocolate, fruits, and vegetables. A child with an eating disorder will often avoid foods like cookies or brownies because they have a reputation for being unhealthy. They will often choose fruits and vegetables because they are viewed as healthy food choices. They also fear that if they allow themselves to eat these 'unhealthy' foods, they will not be able to stop or they will get fat.

This is not true. All kinds of foods should be included in a balanced diet. Snack foods and desserts help with feelings of fullness and satisfaction, which are an important part of the eating experience.

These types of foods should be included in the meal plan one to three times per day. This helps someone with an eating disorder introduce these foods in a structured way and helps challenge their beliefs around these foods.

Q: I'm worried that my son is eating the same types of food every day. There is no variety in his diet. How can I help him incorporate new foods into his meal plan?

A: As your son begins to eat, he will be eating mechanically. Eating mechanically and following a meal plan will feel safe to him and he may not be willing to integrate new foods initially.

Once your child is comfortable with his meal plan, encourage him to introduce a new food item. Work with your child to find out what food he would like to challenge himself with and when he would be willing to do it. Make a plan together and stick to it. Your child may not be ready the first time, but continue to support him and offer these new foods.

What Is Healthy Eating Behavior?

Healthy eating behavior is taken for granted by most people who don't have eating problems, but children and adolescents with eating disorders struggle to eat normally.

Because your child's disordered relationship with food has taken some time to develop, beginning to eat normally may take some time. It requires persistence and patience. Seek help from a professional if needed.

Healthy teenagers eat because they feel hungry, to meet their energy needs, and because they find eating enjoyable. Healthy teenagers eat all kinds of foods — no foods are banned. There is no such thing as a 'good' food or 'bad' food. What is good is moderation, flexibility, and variety. What is bad is excess, compulsivity, rigidity, and lack of options.

Kids are born with an internal regulator that tells them how much food they need at a given time. Sometimes children and teenagers with eating disorders lose touch with their internal regulator. This regulator lets kids know when they are hungry and when they are full. Sometimes teenagers will eat more than usual and other times they will eat less — and that's normal. As children grow, they will eat as much or as little as their bodies need.

Teenager's attitudes, behaviors, and feelings about food and eating are also important to their health and well-being. Children learn about these attitudes from their parents. It is important that you become aware of your own personal attitudes and issues about food and weight. Inaccurate attitudes about food and weight management can lead to dieting, body image concerns, and disordered eating. These kinds of behaviors can put teenagers at risk for an eating disorder.

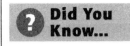

Did You Know...

- Young people may have eaten in a disordered way for so long that they have forgotten what normal, healthy eating is.

- They may have lost their ability to sense hunger and fullness, making it difficult to know how much food their bodies need.

You Can Help...

Even though it may not appear that your children are watching what you do or listening to what you say...they are! This puts you in a great position to be a good role model by eating well-balanced meals and not skipping meals. Don't make comments about your body weight, shape, and size; don't comment about other people's body weight, shape, and size. Don't diet and don't exercise excessively.

HELP FOR NORMALIZING EATING

Whether your child suffers from anorexia nervosa or bulimia nervosa, structured eating is essential. Try helping your child to read and understand this list of suggestions for restoring normal eating behavior. Be patient. Your child may not be ready to try every suggestion right away. As your son or daughter advances in the recovery process, they will start to experiment with different foods and with their sense of being hungry and full.

☐ **More Is Better**
Try eating five to six times per day. Meals and snacks should include foods from all food groups (protein, grains, milk and milk products, fruit, vegetables, fat, and snack foods).

☐ **On Time**
Aim to eat meals and snacks on a time schedule. Try every 2 to 3 hours.

☐ **Back on Track**
If you slip up or miss a meal or snack, just get back on track at the next meal or snack.

☐ **Hunger Pains**
Try not to get overly hungry.

☐ **No More Calories**
Stop counting calories.

☐ **No Restrictions**
Eat according to the meal plan and not according to personal dietary rules or restrictions.

☐ **Dieters Beware**
Try eating with people who are normal eaters and not dieters.

☐ **Going Public**
Practice eating in public places.

☐ **Family Food Time**
Eat with supportive family members and friends in the kitchen or dining room.

☐ **Enjoyable Food**
Throw out all diet products and use regular food instead. Buy foods that are enjoyable to eat.

☐ **No Labels**
Avoid labeling foods as 'good' or 'bad.' Instead, think of flexible and moderate behaviors as good, and excessive and rigid behaviors as bad.

☐ **Flexible Food**
Experiment with foods that haven't been eaten in a while. Make gradual changes instead of drastic changes. Learn to be flexible with food choices.

☐ **Think Positively**
Do not feel guilty. Allow for occasional slip-ups.

☐ **Distract Yourself**
Make a list of things that are relaxing and distracting after eating. This can be especially helpful for struggles with purging.

☐ **Scales Are for Fish**
Throw out the scales — scales focus on weight rather than reaching the goal of healthy eating.

WHAT IS NORMAL EATING?

Ellyn Satter, in her book, *Secrets of Feeding a Healthy Family*, offers these refreshing answers to this frequently asked question.

- Normal eating is going to the table hungry and eating until you are satisfied.

- Normal eating is being able to choose food you like and to get enough of it — not just stopping because you think you should.

- Normal eating is being able to give some thought to your food selection so you get nutritious food, but not being so wary and restrictive that you miss out on enjoyable food.

- Normal eating is sometimes giving yourself permission to eat because you are happy, sad, or bored — or just because it feels good.

- Normal eating is 3 meals a day — or 4 or 5 — or it can be choosing to munch along the way.

- Normal eating is leaving some cookies on the plate because you know you can have some again tomorrow, or eating more now because they taste so wonderful.

- Normal eating is overeating at times; feeling stuffed and uncomfortable. And it can be undereating at times and wishing you had more.

- Normal eating is trusting your body to make up for your mistakes in eating.

- Normal eating takes up some of your time and attention but keeps its place as only one important area of your life.

- In short, normal eating is flexible. It varies in response to your hunger, your schedule, your proximity to food, and your feelings.

What Is a Healthy Weight?

Eating healthy and maintaining a healthy weight are inseparable in restoring the health of a child or adolescent with an eating disorder. These young people are preoccupied with their weight; they are also often misinformed about what a 'healthy' weight means. Achieving and maintaining a healthy weight means being free from disease, being energetic, being strong each day, and being resistant to the negative effects of life's stresses — but not being preoccupied with food.

Weight Factors

The growth and development of each individual child is determined by a number of factors: their genes, their gender, and their energy needs.

Genetics

Your children's genes determine their physical traits; for example, if they will have blue eyes and curly hair. Genes also play an important role in determining your child's body shape, weight, and size. Children have different body types with different healthy weights. Genetics also influence the development of your child through various growth stages — infancy, childhood, and adolescence. As children grow and develop over the years, their weight should naturally increase along with their height. Few children and adolescents develop at exactly the same rate.

Gender

Changes in weight are a normal part of puberty for both girls and boys; this is a time when your child's body changes to that of a young woman or man. Weight gain is a normal part of adolescent growth and development. During this time, your child needs to gain weight.

Boys and girls will experience these weight and height changes differently and at different ages. Girls generally begin puberty earlier than boys, usually between the ages of 7.5 and 12. Boys generally begin puberty between 9.5 and 13.5 years of age. In preparation for puberty, girls gain proportionately more body fat than boys. Young women need more body fat than men. These changes in body composition start as early as puberty.

Energy Needs

Weight may also be affected by the amount of energy your child eats and the amount of energy used. If your child takes in more energy than needed, some weight may be gained. If your daughter or son eats less than their body requires or exercises a lot, then they may lose weight. Small changes in the amount they exercise or eat will not affect weight. The body gets used to these regular kinds of fluctuations. When teenagers eat enough and exercise moderately, they will be at a healthy weight that is right for them.

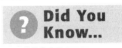 **Did You Know...**

- Because children and adolescents come in all different shapes and sizes, the best weight for your son or daughter is one that is right for their body shape and size.

- There is no one ideal weight that is healthy for all children and adolescents who are of the same height or age. Every child grows and develops in a unique way.

SETPOINT THEORY OF WEIGHT

Your children have inherited an appropriate weight range that the body will move toward naturally as they grow and develop. This is known as the body's setpoint. Setpoint refers to a person's weight when they eat a normal amount of food in a normal way. A person's body will work toward maintaining this weight over the long term.

However, if a person undereats, the body will protect itself by decreasing the amount of energy it burns (its metabolic rate) so that less energy is needed. At the same time, the body will begin to feel more hunger, with increased thoughts about food, accompanied by a desire to eat. This is the body's way of telling a person to eat and restore their natural setpoint weight.

The body will also protect itself from going above the setpoint range by experiencing feelings of fullness or satiety to stop the eating process and it may increase its metabolic rate.

Chaotic eating and weight fluctuations may disturb your child's setpoint.

Weight Fluctuation

Parents need to keep in mind that major weight fluctuations during any stage of growth and development should be regarded with suspicion. Dramatic weight changes can be associated with eating disorders. Weight changes may be the first sign a parent notices and may be the reason why they seek medical attention.

The medical history of your child's growth in height and weight is very important information for your child's assessment and for determining a weight at which your son or daughter's body will function normally. For girls, the weight at which they menstruate regularly is also helpful in determining a healthier weight.

BODY MASS INDEX (BMI)

Body mass index is a calculation that uses a child's weight, height, and age to check on how the child is growing. In children and teens, BMI is used to determine whether a young person is underweight, overweight, or at risk for being overweight. As children grow and develop, their body fat changes. Girls and boys differ in their body fat as they mature. This is why BMI for children is based on gender and age.

The best way to determine your child's BMI is to have your doctor do it for you. That way, you'll know that the number is accurate, and your doctor can discuss the results with you and your child. There are special BMI charts (there's one for boys and one for girls) to help your doctor compare your child to a group of healthy boys or girls in the same age group.

This functional weight is used only as an estimate and should be expected to change as your child grows and develops with age. Questions or concerns regarding your child's weight should be discussed with your child's health-care professional.

Physical Activity

A healthy lifestyle includes eating normally, maintaining a healthy weight, and exercising moderately. Exercise is good for the body and the soul. Exercise helps make the heart, muscles, and bones stronger and also helps reduce the risk of many diseases. It can help your son or daughter better manage the stresses of life and may increase their self-esteem.

However, teenagers struggling with an eating disorder may use exercise in a way that is not compatible with their health. They may become dependent on exercise to change their shape or to lose weight or to get rid of food they have eaten.

If exercise is not playing a helpful role, help your daughter or son to understand their motivation for exercising. Physical activity may need to be limited or initially eliminated when helping your child to get well. Your health-care professional may help you and your child identify when it is safe to introduce physical activity.

When reintroducing activity, it is important to start slowly and choose activities that are social, such as team sports. Setting time and distance limits are also important to keep your child from overexercising or exercising for the wrong reasons. Their meal plan may also need to be increased to ensure they are getting the energy back that was lost during exercise.

Athletic girls who don't get enough nutrition and who don't have their menstrual periods may develop weakened bones. Inappropriate amounts of food, low body fat, and the stress of intense sport may cause their bodies to not produce enough of the hormone called estrogen, which is important for regular menstrual periods and for keeping bones strong. These weakened bones may lead to osteoporosis. This may be irreversible.

Healthy nutrition and maintenance of a healthy weight are needed to have normal menstrual periods and, ultimately, to keep bones growing to their highest potential.

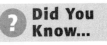
Did You Know...

• Some girls who play competitive sports or exercise excessively are at risk for a problem called the female athlete triad.

• The female athlete triad includes disordered eating, lack of a menstrual period for more than 3 consecutive months, and osteoporosis.

MENU IDEAS FOR HEALTHY TEENAGERS

To make eating meals and snacks more enjoyable for your child, consider experimenting with these menu ideas, alternating them, and adding your own family touches to them. Ask your child to participate in the menu planning process.

Breakfast

- Bagel or English muffin with peanut butter, a piece of fruit or glass of orange juice and glass of milk.

- Oatmeal made with milk, a piece of fruit and a glass of juice.

- Pancakes or waffles with butter and maple syrup, a piece of fruit, and a glass of milk.

- Cereal with milk, a piece of fruit, and yogurt.

- Toast with margarine/butter, scrambled eggs, fresh fruit, and a glass of milk.

- Yogurt, fruit, granola, and toast with cream cheese or peanut butter.

- Bacon or sausage, eggs, toast, and a glass of milk.

- Congee rice or rice porridge made plain and served with a variety of salty, pickled, and stir-fried dishes or served with chicken, pork, fish, or shrimp.

- Pho (Vietnamese) noodle soup with either beef or chicken.

Lunch

- Sandwich with meat, tuna, eggs, or cheese, mayonnaise or margarine/butter, and vegetables (e.g., cucumbers, lettuce, tomatoes), a piece of fruit or box of raisins, yogurt, and cookies.

- Pizza with cheese and vegetables and/or meat, and milk/juice/soda pop.

- Beef, chicken, or veggie burger with condiments (e.g., mayonnaise, ketchup, lettuce, and tomato), french fries, and milk/juice/soda pop.

- Submarine sandwich with meat, cheese, and vegetables, salad with dressing, cookies, and glass of milk.

Dinner

- Meat (chicken, pork, fish or beef), baked potato, vegetables with margarine/ butter/oil, milk, and ice cream.

- Stir-fry with meat or tofu, rice, and vegetables made with oil, milk and cookies.

- Pasta with tomato/meat sauce, salad with dressing, garlic bread, milk, and dessert.

- Pizza with cheese, vegetables, and/or meat, salad with dressing, milk, and fruit.

- Fajitas with meat, beans, and/or cheese, milk, and dessert.

- Chili with meat and/or beans and vegetables, bread, salad with dressing, milk, and dessert.

Snacks

- Granola bars, cereal bars
- Pudding
- Yogurt
- Cookies
- Ice cream or sherbet
- Crackers and cheese
- Muffins
- Cereal and milk

- Fruit
- Bagel or English muffin with cream cheese or peanut butter
- Pizza
- Chocolate bars
- Chips or pretzels or popcorn
- Vegetables and dip
- Nuts or trail mix

Q: My child is going to camp for a couple of weeks this summer. How can I ensure that she is getting enough nutrition?

A: The first step is to learn about the camp's daily routine, meal structure, and menu offerings. This will help you and your daughter plan how her current eating pattern and foods can be incorporated into the new routine. Discuss your child's struggles with the camp director and the camp doctor or nurse. It may be necessary to request that your child is monitored while eating to ensure she is completing her meals and snacks. Most camps will allow children to bring along their favorite snacks. Ensure your daughter brings snacks she likes to eat.

CHAPTER 14

Coping with Lapses and Relapses

During the course of your child's recovery from an eating disorder, both lapses and relapses can be expected. Though the thought of a lapse or a relapse can be frightening to parents, be assured that they are a normal part of recovery. They are part of the process of change. The road to recovering from an eating disorder is long, and it is the lessons learned along the way that lead to successful recovery.

There are a number of reasons adolescents with eating disorders may experience a lapse or a relapse. In many cases, the eating disorder thoughts are so intense that it becomes very difficult for them to fight back. In other instances, something may happen that is experienced as stressful. Returning to former eating patterns and behaviors can be a manner of coping. Often young people who have faced stress have found comfort in their eating disorder and have employed it as a coping mechanism.

Remember that each day is a new day. What happened yesterday cannot be changed. What your child chooses to do today and in following days can be changed, though. Bear with the lapses and relapses. Your patience and support will help your child to recover.

What Are Lapses and Relapses?

During the process of recovery, a child or adolescent with an eating disorder will have several lapses. This is normal. Lapses are to be expected. Relapses are also normal during the process of change.

? Did You Know...

• Research shows that patients who are discharged from an inpatient program when they are at 80% of their progress or target weight have a 75% chance of being readmitted to hospital.

• Adolescents who are discharged when they are at 85% or more of their progress or target weight have a 75% chance of not being readmitted to hospital.

Stages of Recovery

Although the stages of change along the road to recovery appear to be straightforward, most adolescents recovering from an eating disorder find that they slip back and forth between these stages of change. Don't be discouraged by this slippage — lapses and relapses occur. From each attempt to change, your child becomes better prepared for the next effort. Don't let the first lapse or relapse become an excuse for not trying again.

- Precontemplation (resisting change)
- Contemplation (thinking about change)
- Preparation (planning to change)
- Action (changing)
- Maintenance (maintaining changes)
- Termination (moving on)

Lapses

For adolescents with an eating disorder, a lapse occurs occasionally when the old eating disorder thoughts and behaviors overpower their ability to fight back. For example, a young woman who is doing well restoring her weight on her own one day feels that she cannot follow her meal plan and skips both her dinner and her evening snack. The next morning she resumes her program by eating her breakfast.

Relapses

A relapse occurs when children or adolescents with an eating disorder are no longer able to maintain the changes they've made. The mind-set associated with the eating disorder returns, and the child or adolescent relapses into disordered eating behaviors. For example, a young woman with bulimia nervosa has been having her meals at regular times for the several months, which has helped her to reduce her desire to binge. When the thoughts and feelings of her eating disorder return, she is no longer able to control her desire to binge. She starts to binge in the evenings and resumes her old pattern of restricting during the day.

Q: My 15-year-old daughter is struggling with bulimia nervosa. The past week has been really good. She's been eating all her meals with us and has been spending time with her sister after meals to keep herself busy. Last night, her sister wasn't home and right after dinner she went up to the bathroom and I could hear her throwing up. I'm scared that she's going to start this cycle all over again. What can we do to help her?

A: Talk with your daughter about what you've noticed. Let her know in a caring way that you are concerned that she may be starting her binging cycle again. Find out if there is anything in particular that she feels led her to binge, and whether there is anything that could be done to make a change so that she doesn't feel tempted again. It is possible that she may have found it difficult to be on her own after dinner last night. It is unlikely that her sister can be with her after every meal, but perhaps there is someone else in your family who could spend time with her after meals to help keep her mind off of binging. Explore with her what she feels would be supportive to her.

Protecting against Lapses and Relapses

While lapses and relapses are bound to happen, you can minimize them using the following tools.

Know Your Environment

Be aware of your child's environment. Are there stressful elements to the environment? If so, what are they? Could any of these elements be changed?

A common experience for adolescents with eating disorders is the anxiety associated with having to eat lunch at school, particularly when the lunch they have may be much larger than what their friends are eating. If teens are feeling anxious about this even before they get into the situation, there is a good chance that once they are at lunch with their friends they will choose not to eat their lunch. Since this can have an impact on their recovery, it is necessary to think about what can be changed in the situation to make them feel more comfortable. In this instance, it might mean finding a different group of friends to eat with, who eat a regular lunch, or meeting a parent or relative for lunch until they feel more comfortable.

Preplanning with your teen about ways to cope with the stress, other than through eating disordered behaviors, can be helpful. This is an opportunity to start countering some of your child's unhealthy eating patterns with healthier behaviors. If your son or daughter binges when stressed, you can work with them to establish other things they could do to cope with feelings, such as going for a walk, writing in a journal, or calling a friend.

Work with your child to determine what situations they feel may be difficult for them, and then brainstorm around how to make changes in order to create a more supportive environment.

CASE STUDY Susan

At Susan's next clinic visit, she found out that her weight was down and she was medically unstable. There as no choice…she needed to be readmitted to hospital. Susan started to cry when she got the news. "There is no way I am going into the hospital again. I have a math test tomorrow…I can't miss it! You can't make me come into the hospital. I hate all of you…" She refused to be admitted.

Both her parents and the team told her she had no choice. She would have to be admitted against her will. She settled down when the security guards arrived. She agreed to go voluntarily.

Once Susan was settled, her father went back to talk to her team. He couldn't understand why she had relapsed. Everything had been going pretty well. The child psychiatrist explained that lapses and relapses were common.

"Sometimes young people with eating disorders find a place in their illness where they can just coast along. Their weight is high enough that they can continue as outpatients and avoid admission. Things at home, school,

and friends are all okay. They can manage their life, stay underweight, and avoid hospitalization. They know everyone wants them to gain weight, but this is easy to ignore, because there is no real cost to them. Under these circumstances, there is no motivation to get better from the eating disorder. In fact, the teen may even be convinced that the eating disorder is helpful and seems to be holding things together. There is nothing distressing going on in the teen's life to help move them out of denial.

"In the Day Treatment Program," her psychiatrist continued, "Susan started to get better and that was frightening to her. The voice of the eating disorder was loud in her head, pointing out how 'fat' she was getting. Susan panicked and lost the weight.

"The best thing everyone can do is stay calm and empathic…but be firm! We have to support Susan as she becomes medically stable and then she can be discharged back to the Day Treatment Program."

continued on page 239

Develop Countering Techniques

Learning to counter unhealthy thoughts and behaviors with more positive thoughts and behaviors is an important tool for both adolescents and parents. Using alternate activities and coping phrases may help.

Alternative Activities: going for a walk, reading a book, listening to music, watching television, or calling a friend instead of engaging in an eating disorder behavior, such as excessive exercising or binging.

Coping Phrases: such phrases as "I can do it," "I have so much to look forward to," and "It's okay" can be rehearsed either internally or out loud, to help your child through difficult times.

Reward Your Child

During the course of recovering from an eating disorder, both small steps and big steps should be rewarded. For example, for an adolescent with anorexia nervosa, eating breakfast is a big deal. Likewise, for an adolescent with bulimia nervosa, delaying a binge episode by an hour is also a significant accomplishment.

EATING DISORDER TRIGGERS

Recognizing what triggers a lapse or relapse can help you to spot difficulties that may come up. For example, if your child is going to be starting Grade 9 at a new high school, you may anticipate that this will be a stressful time.

The following is a list of triggers that have been identified by adolescents with eating disorders. Triggers for each adolescent will be different.

- Starting a new school or returning to a school after a long absence
- School marks, tests, or exams
- Traveling away from home (going on a trip or going to camp)
- Peer pressure
- Issues with a friend or a group of friends
- Being bullied
- Loss of a family member or loss of a family pet
- Family stress
- A family vacation

Q: My son James is 13 years old and was diagnosed with anorexia nervosa 18 months ago. He has been out of the hospital for one year now and has been doing well. I'm starting to get worried because he looks as though he is losing weight. His clothes seem much looser on him. What's going on?

A: Take some time to notice what has been going on for James lately. Does he seem to be eating his meals? Has he been exercising? Has he withdrawn from his friends or from family? Talk with James about how he feels he has been doing. Explore with him whether there have been any recent stresses for him. Is there anything that may have triggered his return to his old eating behaviors? Work with James to determine what he thinks would be helpful to him to get him back on track.

A reward for such an accomplishment can be as simple as telling your daughter or son that they have done a good job. You see that they are working hard. Rewards do not need to be material. Give them a hug to let them know you are supporting them.

Adolescents may choose to reward themselves with things like an outing with friends or with an extra hour of a favorite activity. Families may choose to reward larger steps, such as eating 'phobic' foods again or not binging for a week.

HELP FOR COPING WITH LAPSES AND RELAPSES

As parents, it is difficult to watch your teen experience a lapse or relapse. However, there are many things that you can do to support your child.

- Talk to your daughter or son and ask what kind of help they would like from you. Don't be surprised if they say they are doing fine and don't need any help; they may be once again contemplating whether they are ready to give up their eating disorder.

- Bear with your child's lack of readiness to change. Most often parents are ready for the action stage of change long before their children are. However, your child needs to be motivated to make change, and the change can only come from within. As parents you will need to encourage your child to keep working hard to fight the eating disorder, but you cannot win the battle for your son or daughter. In order for change to last, children and adolescents need to be motivated for their own reasons to keep the eating disorder out of their life.

- Talk with your treatment team. They will be able to assist and support your child and family.

- Of utmost importance is to remain calm. Rest assured that your child will get through this lapse or relapse and will continue on with recovery. Remind yourself that the process of change takes time.

CHAPTER 15

Making the Transition from the Adolescent to the Adult Treatment System

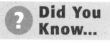 **Did You Know...**

- Adolescents making the transition to the adult system will now be recognized as a young adults.

- They will have all the rights society grants to adults, including the decision to accept or reject treatment.

Adolescents and their families receiving treatment for eating disorders always hope this treatment will be their last and that they will not require further help. Unfortunately, some adolescents continue to struggle with their eating disorder into adulthood and require care in the adult treatment system. They will move from a pediatric health-care system to an adult health-care system.

Pediatric and adult health-care professionals work together with the young person and the family to help make this transition successful. A successful transition involves careful planning about who will handle the person's care and careful choosing among the treatment options available in the community. During this time of transition, health-care professionals will support a patient's growing sense of independence and encourage young people to take responsibility for their own health care. Health-care professionals also offer families information on what to expect during this transition.

While facing this transition, parents and adolescents with eating disorders naturally have many questions.

At What Age Does this Transition Usually Occur?

Adolescents will need to be transferred to the adult system if it appears that they will not make a full recovery by the time they reach a predetermined age called "the age of transition".

Age of Transition

The needs of adolescents differ widely depending on their age and their level of emotional development. In general, your health-care system or treatment setting will designate a specific age for the transition of adolescents (for example, some centers require that transition to the adult health-care system occur by18 years). The exact age at which this occurs depends on where the patient is receiving services. Depending on where you live, there may be a brief period of overlap in services during this transitional period.

Early Transition

In some situations, this decision is made earlier, especially when the illness is severe and has the potential to continue for a longer period of time. Some treatment services may move adolescents into the adult system a bit early if it is clear that they require ongoing treatment, are unlikely to benefit from continued treatment in the pediatric system, and are ready to work with an older group of co-patients.

If the young person requires inpatient treatment, then ideally a member of the adult team will meet with them and, if possible, the family, to discuss the needs of the patient, what the adult system can offer, and how this might be different from the adolescent system. This process will vary from program to program across the country and in other countries.

> **? Did You Know…**
>
> • A factor to be considered in the decision to transfer care to the adult system is the adolescent's overall stage of development.
>
> • Young people who are more emotionally mature may fit in better with adult treatment services.

How Does this Transition Proceed?

The pediatric treatment team explores how to best prepare for a possible transition to adult treatment programs with the adolescent and the family.

Coordinator

The pediatric team will often designate someone to help coordinate the young person's transition. This health-care professional will contact the adult treatment center to discuss various treatment options that will best meet the needs of the young person. Often, the coordinator from the pediatric team and a representative from the adult treatment program will meet with the young person and the family to develop a transition plan. During these joint meetings, the young person can ask questions about the various treatment options and raise any concerns about leaving a program designed for teens and entering a new and unfamiliar system.

Transition Report

When a plan has been made, the pediatric team will write a transition report that can be forwarded to your family doctor and other local service providers involved in the young person's ongoing care. The pediatric health-care professionals may also provide information to families about available support services. Some families find it helpful to ask questions about the adult treatment system and the changes expected to occur before their child exits the pediatric system.

Care Plan

Once the decision has been made to transfer the young person, the pediatric team will recommend to the adolescent and family that they meet with a member of the adult eating disorder program to develop a plan for the individual's ongoing care. This plan should include a discussion about what available resources might be useful to them. For example, it may be clear that the young person has gained back some weight but is suffering from binging and purging. Individuals with this type of problem might be better suited for outpatient or day hospital treatment.

Limitations

Specialized adult eating disorder programs often do not have the capacity to provide ongoing care or individual therapy for the young adult with an eating disorder. These programs may only have the capacity to make periodic assessments of the young adult's status and make recommendations for specific forms of care — for example, admission to the day hospital program or the inpatient program. Most adult eating disorder programs have little or no capacity for emergency admission. The care plan for transfer almost never includes a transfer of an inpatient from the adolescent hospital to the adult hospital.

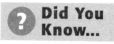

Did You Know...

• Transition to adult care is most successful when young adults share responsibility for the decision with the health-care professionals and the family.

• When they are assessed, family involvement is strongly encouraged, though the decision ultimately rests with the young adult as to whether they want their family involved or not.

What Are the Differences Between the Systems?

Both the pediatric and the adult systems share many approaches and common goals in providing a mixture of medical, psychological, and nutritional treatments designed as much as possible to fit the needs of a given person.

Adult Responsibility

In the adolescent system, parents or other adults are an important part of the decision-making process with respect to medical treatment. Efforts are made to work together with adolescents whenever possible in order to engage them in their treatment. While many young adults with eating disorders will be eager to continue with their treatment, some will decide that they are no longer interested in treatment once they have control over their treatment decisions.

In the adult system, the decisions regarding treatment for an eating disorder almost always rest with the young adult. While this varies depending on where you live, in general, adults are viewed as being in charge of decisions about their medical treatment unless it can be conclusively shown that they do not appreciate or understand the situation they are in. For parents who have had a significant role in decision-making for their child, it may be surprising how much autonomy the adult system affords for decision-making, even for very ill individuals.

Voluntary Treatment

An enormous distinction about such decisions is that treatment in the adult system is usually voluntary. An involuntary intervention in the adult system is considered to be 'management' as opposed to 'treatment'.

Confidentiality

Another important difference between the adolescent and the adult systems is the extent of communication between the health-care professionals and the family. Without consent from the young adult with an eating disorder, health-care professionals cannot even talk with families about the young adult's care, even if they are living with their family or their family is otherwise actively involved in their lives.

? Did You Know...

• While you may clearly see your child as not able to make decisions, the authorities charged with making such decisions may not agree with you.

• While the adult system does everything possible to encourage young adults to involve their families, in the end, young adults will make their own treatment decisions.

While the legal and ethical limitations of confidentiality will vary depending on the laws and the location of the health-care system, in most jurisdictions, mental health information cannot be communicated without the consent of the patient.

However, health-care professionals encourage young adults with eating disorders to speak honestly and openly with their families. If young adults no longer wish their treatment team to speak with their family, it can be difficult for families who are used to having ongoing regular contact with the adolescent team. This makes it very important to try to maintain good relationships between the young person and family.

Serious Medical Problems

Another difference between treatment of adolescents and adults is how serious medical problems are addressed.

When adolescents are assessed as needing care for an eating disorder, they are typically treated in eating disorder units by health-care professionals specially trained in dealing with the specific acute medical and emotional aspects of these disorders.

In contrast, when young adults are assessed in an outpatient office or hospital emergency department for medical complications, they are often transferred to the care of a general internal medicine service, intensive care unit, emergency department, or family medicine ward, as appropriate. In the adult system, an emergency admission does not lead to an automatic entry into the eating disorder program intended for adults who are medically stable and voluntarily wish to pursue treatment for their eating symptoms.

The medical treatment of eating disorders also varies between adolescents and adults due to differences in medical problems experienced by individuals at different stages of the illness. Adolescents with eating disorders are typically identified closer to the beginning of their illness when their bodies are still growing and developing, which may increase the risk of developing severe and long-term medical problems. These potentially serious problems require very careful medical monitoring.

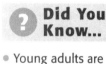

Did You Know...

• Young adults are more likely to have had the illness longer and their bodies are, therefore, more adapted to being starved.

• Consequently, they appear more physically stable.

Adults are almost never forced into hospital against their will, and when this does happen, it happens at much lower weights than tolerated in the adolescent system. These differences are often very troubling for parents who may not be familiar with these differences.

CASE STUDY Jessica

When I turned 17½ years old, my eating disorder treatment team started to talk to me about "transitioning" to the adult health-care system. I was filled with emotions…terrified, sad and angry!

I loved my dietitian. She was the first person who really understood me and helped me with my eating. It was hard to imagine not having my therapist to talk to. I had worked so hard over the past year…I felt so connected. And then there was my pediatrician…she wouldn't let me get away with anything! I counted on her for that.

I didn't feel ready to be treated like an adult. I think my parents were also concerned about this transition. They were so used to being involved in my treatment at the pediatric eating disorder program. They worried about not being active participants in my treatment in the adult system.

The process of transition was very hard! The pediatric team was firm in their kind way. They helped us through the process.

I remember getting really angry with the team…I felt like they just wanted to get rid of me! My therapist helped me work through my feelings of abandonment and rejection. The entire team supported me through these difficult times.

The team organized a joint meeting with members from the adult eating disorder team. Me, my parents, my pediatric eating disorder team, and the members of the adult eating disorder team were all there. It was scary…but it was very helpful. Most importantly, they explained their program, my role, and my parents' role. They answered all our questions.

I actually needed the whole 6 months to get used to the idea of leaving the pediatric eating disorder program. During that time, I decided that my parents would be part of my recovery. I consented to have them involved with my ongoing treatment in the adult health-care system.

continued on page 252

What Problems Can Happen During this Transition?

While this transition often goes smoothly, sometimes there are disagreements between young adults, their families, and their treatment teams. What happens when the transition is not smooth and there are differences of opinion?

Extent of Treatment

Most young adults welcome having increased control over their own treatment and will typically choose to exercise this freedom. However, parents may react with horror to the notion that their involvement in treatment may be sharply curtailed because the decision-making power now lies with their daughter or son. This is usually related to fears that they will die if not held in treatment against their will or a belief that the young adult is simply not experienced or mature enough to make sensible treatment decisions.

Maturity

Most of the adolescents who make the transition from the pediatric to the adult system have been in treatment for some time. Because of their illness, they may not have had the usual teenage experience of gradually taking increased responsibility for their decisions. They may believe that they cannot make good decisions about other areas in their life, such as school, work, and relationships. Some young people believe that the eating disorder is the only aspect of their life they can control. They may have great difficulties making decisions about entering and staying in treatment, especially when their eating disorder defines who they are.

Some young adults, transferred into the adult system, certainly do have difficulty making sound decisions about many things that may not be related to their eating disorder. They may need considerable help in developing this capacity. Often this process is not complete until the young adult eventually makes a substantial recovery, after which time families routinely comment that they cannot believe how rapidly the young person completes the process of 'growing up'.

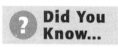

Did You Know...

• The most common area of conflict between young adults with eating disorders and their parent is when the parents think that the young adult needs more treatment and the young adult disagrees.

Isolation

Many young adults are conscious of the fact that their friends who do not have eating disorders are becoming more independent and are moving on with their lives. Most young adults with a serious eating disorder will eventually feel like they have been left behind. Naturally, the eating disorder serves as a 'brake' on such catch-ups, and usually limits the extent to which a young person can make progress in other areas of life. It can take some years for young people to understand this and connect their lack of progress in their life to their eating disorder.

Changing Roles

The role of parents in the adult system can be confusing to them and to their child. In some cases, parent and child develop a strong sense of partnership about combating the illness that they carry into the adult system. Some young adults who have experienced many involuntary admissions will have developed an 'us versus them' attitude and view not only parents but most adults as somehow in opposition to their life goals. Other young adults simply take some time to recognize that they are allowed to ask their parents for help, and that asking for help is an acceptable adult behavior. Some are so delayed in their social development that they cannot even consider taking on more responsibility for themselves and become very passive and unable to make any decisions.

Another common concern for parents is their own sense of inadequacy and failure when their child needs ongoing care. Parents may feel that they didn't try hard enough, or that efforts they had made were somehow sabotaged. Parents with a son or daughter who is ambivalent and reluctant to engage in treatment may feel a sense of loss based on their previous active involvement with the adolescent treatment team. Similar to pediatric health-care professionals, adult eating disorder professionals make every effort to convey to families that they are not to blame for their child's illness.

Dependence

Some young people may find it very difficult to cope with the eating disorder once they leave the pediatric system. These young adults may appear much younger than their chronological age, or seem to have difficulty in making any type of decision on their own. Parents may feel very concerned that their children are being given too much responsibility before they are ready.

Others may feel secure entering the adult system because it provides them with a safe place where they can control their eating behaviors. Once there, they may not want to leave because they become emotionally connected to the health-care professionals and become accustomed to the structure and safety provided by the treatment program. Unfortunately, it may take several admissions for some young people to transfer what they are learning in the program to their everyday life.

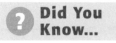

Did You Know...

• Young adults commonly become very attached to the adolescent treatment team and may be terrified to be transferred to the adult system.

Help for Making the Transition

The first and most important thing for parents to remember is that their child has made a significant transition once they have entered the adult system. While some parents may have grave reservations about their children's ability to manage, the focus must shift toward teaching these young adults basic skills to manage their lives.

Develop a New Adult Relationship

Dealing with a young adult's belief that they 'know everything' and are all-powerful can be trying at times. Try focusing on the type of relationship that you eventually wish to have with your child. Will it be characterized by a respectful adult dialog or threats and blame? Do you see a child who is permanently dependent on you? The type of relationship you want should guide your actions. You will often find yourself leading by example, trying hard to demonstrate what a healthy adult response would be. Efforts to confront the young person's control over the eating disorder often fail.

Experiment

Young adults who appear to be making poor decisions may respond to the 'experiment' approach. Should your daughter or son tell you that they are going to 'try it on my own' for a while, think about asking them to set some goals. For example, what type of result at what time would mean that the 'experiment' of 'trying it on my own' was a success or failure? With this type of approach, letting the young adult set the ground rules will produce better results because it means they are taking responsibility for their future.

It is appropriate to set some limits around such experiments. For example, you might say you will accept their experiment as long as they are seeing their family doctor regularly for medical monitoring. Or, you may tell a young adult who is binging that within a certain period of time any food taken from the family must be replaced. These limits act as safety nets, both for the young adult and the rest of the family, allowing for some independent exploration while protecting against life-threatening consequences.

Support Independence

We strongly recommend that parents of young adults who have been ill for some time work hard toward promoting independence as being healthy and appropriate given their age. It is enormously challenging when your child chooses to separate from you by making a treatment decision with which you disagree. However, it is usually a mistake to view efforts to be more independent as willful or 'bad'. Framing such efforts in this way may actually result in the young person deliberately avoiding advice and support from parents — just when they may need it the most.

Seek Support for Yourself

Parents may need support during this transition to deal with feelings of hopelessness, helplessness, and abandonment. This support may come from the adult treatment team, if your child has given permission for you to be involved, from other sources of professional support, or from parent support groups. The most important thing is to not lose hope.

WORSHEET

TRANSITION CHECKLIST

Here is a list of suggestions for parents as they help their young adult's transition from the pediatric health-care to the adult health-care system.

Activity

☐ Talk about this process early. Transition is a process that should occur gradually over time and include you, your child, and the pediatric and adult health-care teams.

☐ Encourage your son or daughter to be actively involved in the transition process.

☐ Understand your child's thoughts and feelings about taking responsibility for their own eating disorder care.

☐ Use the treatment team to help you and your child decide on your child's ongoing treatment needs, which health-care professionals your child will need to see, who will make the referrals, and who will help coordinate this process.

☐ Be clear about which health-care professionals will be involved in taking over your child's health care once in the adult health-care system.

☐ Support meetings between the pediatric health-care professionals, the adult health-care professionals, you, and your child.

☐ Identify the goals of treatment in the new health-care setting. Define the new roles and responsibilities of the young adult, parents, and treatment team.

☐ Encourage your child to talk to the adult health-care professionals and to ask questions.

☐ Talk with your son or daughter about their ongoing health care needs for their eating disorder — what skills is your child able to perform, what skills does your child need to learn, and what skills does your child require assistance with?

☐ Help prepare and educate your child for the adult health-care system. Make certain your child knows about their past medical history, current medications, and allergies. Some young adults carry this information in their wallet or purse.

☐ Encourage your son or daughter to schedule and prepare for their own medical appointments.

☐ Discuss medical insurance coverage. Provide young adults with insurance information (medical insurance carriers and numbers) and encourage them to carry this information.

☐ Review how to access your child's medical records.

☐ Review how to get prescriptions filled and refilled.

WORKSHEET

☐ Talk about how your child will get to and from the treatment appointments.

☐ Make sure your child is aware of the danger signs associated with the eating disorder. Develop a plan of action with your child should any of these danger signs occur.

☐ Ensure your son or daughter has emergency telephone numbers with them at all times should they need them.

☐ Make sure they understand that you are there to help and support them, as always.

☐ Model informed and proactive health care. Parents are role models for children at all ages.

What Are the Chances of a Young Adult Recovering?

Many parents are naturally concerned about what will happen to their adolescent if they have not made a good recovery by the time they become adults.

On the one hand, parents need to be aware that the average time for recovery is approximately 6 years, and that children who have not made a recovery in the first 2 years of their illness are likely to remain ill for some time before they get better. Sadly, some people who suffer from an eating disorder will die. Most of the deaths occur either in the first 2 years or after 15 years of suffering with the illness.

On the other hand, parents need to know there is good chance for recovery, no matter how long in duration or how severe the illness. There is no way to tell what route your child will take to recovery; but do know that the adult health-care professionals will certainly commit to traveling with you and your young adult until you all reach that destination. Although it may take some time, most young adults make a good recovery.

The Struggle of My Life
A Patient's Story

I USED TO BELIEVE THE CLICHÉ THAT "A WOMAN CAN NEVER BE too rich or too thin." After experiencing many years of suffering with anorexia nervosa, I now know that this isn't true! When I hear people say that they have "gained weight" or joke about their desire to be a "little anorexic," I use all of my self-restraint to hold back a comment. I know only too well that being a "little anorexic," like being a "little pregnant," isn't possible. There is only anorexia nervosa. It may be moderate or it may severe, but it is anorexia nervosa. I know all about anorexia nervosa because I suffered with this disorder. This is my story of succumbing to the disorder and my recovery.

I knew something was wrong...

I was 14 years old and about to start high school when I first started to show signs and symptoms of an eating disorder. I had always been a good eater and maintained a normal, healthy weight. I now had to adjust to a new environment with lots of new students and teachers at high school. I was so busy that I was unaware of any weight loss. By the time I went to my doctor for my yearly check-up, I had lost 10 pounds without really noticing it. My doctor was not concerned and attributed the weight loss to my new high-school lifestyle and said, "She is still within a normal range for her height." He left it at that.

> I know only too well that being a "little anorexic," like being a "little pregnant," isn't possible.

By the time I was 15, I realized something was wrong. While I was not drastically underweight, I was conscious of the fact that I never "pigged out" like my other friends. I ate in a very controlled way. I was uncertain about what was going on and was not sure if I might have an eating disorder. Eating disorders were not something you discussed openly. If I really had lost a drastic amount of weight in a short time, my parents would have noticed. But the change in my weight was gradual and that made it harder to detect.

My parents and I always had open lines of communication, but life was busy. We barely saw one another between school and other activities. I was always a diligent student and a model daughter. My parents took pride in having such a "low-maintenance" child. I thought I was "eating funny" but wasn't sure how to broach the subject. Probably a part of me was defensive and protective of my strange eating patterns. It was my habit and part of my routine. While it was strange, I felt it had become me.

While I was not drastically underweight, I was conscious of the fact that I never "pigged out" like my other friends.

By the time I was 16, I rapidly spiraled beyond the point of no return. I was weighing myself on my bathroom scale multiple times a day. I was rigidly monitoring my food intake. I was swimming laps almost daily. I was always "on the go." In fact, the family joke was that if I had to go anywhere, I would run instead of walk. All of this was in an effort to control my weight. At the time, my parents, friends, and I seemed to be blind to all of the warning signs. However, hindsight is 20/20.

At the same time, many people reinforced my behavior by telling me how envious they were of my self-discipline with respect to my "healthy" eating habits and daily exercise regime. I took pride in the fact that salespeople complimented me on my small clothing size. I felt unique for the first time and I enjoyed that.

Up until I turned 17, I was able to starve myself without anyone challenging me. My friends were suspicious, but they felt I would resent them if they spoke to my parents behind my back. I was always a small person, and while my family knew I was thin, they didn't think I was ill. Furthermore, my parents did not have firsthand knowledge of anyone with an eating disorder. They were oblivious to the warning signs and symptoms that I had been exhibiting for years. After a third consecutive year of weight loss, my doctor made a joke about "the food in my house not being to Tammy's liking." By that time, I had lost so much weight that I had stopped getting my menstrual period. I chose to withhold that piece of information.

My disorder is finally detected...

The following month, I went to an overnight camp in the United States, where I had a summer job as a lifeguard. Six weeks into the summer, the camp director confronted me with his concerns that I might have an eating disorder. He was so worried that he called my parents. Not only had I lost 10 pounds, but I was also neglecting my responsibilities at the camp. While I was angry that my parents were called, part of me was relieved that I didn't have to hide anymore. I was tired, weak, and hungry.

My parents were shocked and confused when they received the phone call from camp. They dropped everything and immediately came to pick me up. We drove home and no one said a word for the entire 7-hour ride. The following morning we went to our local children's hospital for an emergency eating disorder assessment. I was considered to be "severely ill" and immediately admitted to the hospital. My family and I were suddenly thrust into a scary new world that we never knew existed. My heart rate was critically low. I found myself in a hospital gown hooked up to a heart monitor on the adolescent eating disorder ward. I was terrified and overwhelmed by everything that happened to me over the previous 24 hours.

I was considered to be "severely ill" and immediately admitted to the hospital. My family and I were suddenly thrust into a scary new world that we never knew existed.

My mom repeatedly asked me why I hadn't told her or my father that I was not eating. She was also upset with my friends for not telling any adults that I had a problem. Most of all, she blamed herself and my father. After all, they lived with me and never saw how strange my behavior had become. I felt guilty and I kept crying and apologizing for the mess I had caused them.

My first few days in the hospital are a blur of nurses, doctors, and tears of self-pity. While I was grappling with my own emotions and the reality of my new situation, my parents and three sisters busied themselves with reading everything they could about eating disorders. They went to the bookstore and bought every book they could get their hands on. After the initial shock wore off, they did their best to support me to get well as soon as possible. The doctors reassured my family and me that we were in the best place and that the hospitalization would help me get well. This was comforting to my parents, who just wanted their "old Tammy" back.

From the first day of that hospitalization, I was angry and resentful about being admitted. After all, I was a teenager and saw myself as invincible. The last place I wanted to spend my summer vacation was on an adolescent eating disorder unit. I was ready to admit that I had a problem, but I refused to acknowledge how serious it was. On the outside, I played "compliant patient," but on the inside, I was very confused.

Learning the tricks of the trade...

Later that summer, I was discharged from the hospital. I was more entrenched in my anorexia nervosa than I had been a month earlier. During my hospital admission, I spent a lot of time with other adolescents who suffered with an eating disorder. I had learned new "tricks of the trade" from my fellow patients. I found myself in a strange world of competitive eating disordered teens who had no real desire to get well. Most of the teens were also there against their will and did not understand the seriousness of their illness. I went home filled with unhealthy information and adamant that I was *not* going to gain any more weight. I had my family convinced that I was going to put all my efforts into getting well. Yet, I had joined an elite subculture of self-destructive teens with eating disorders...my previous goals and priorities fell by the wayside.

My family had very little knowledge about eating disorders prior to my diagnosis. They had seen me struggle in the hospital, but they had no idea of what lay ahead of them. My family welcomed me home with open arms. My arrival home began with great optimism and hopes that life would return to normal.

However, things did not happen as we had expected. My parents were overprotective, and as a result, I felt stifled. Fights erupted daily. The eating disorder team at the children's hospital told my parents that it would be acceptable for them to monitor my eating. They took this job very seriously. I could not handle the constant supervision. My parents also worried about me more than they ever had before. I had no freedom. In my parent's eyes, I had become vulnerable and sickly. They had great difficulty letting me out of their sight. I was also trying to adjust to my last year in high school. This was a struggle since I felt that I had no control over my own life. As well, everyone in my school had heard about my hospitalization, and I felt like I was being treated differently. I didn't want sympathy from everyone. I was so frustrated with all of the changes to my life.

> *My parents were overprotective, and as a result, I felt stifled. Fights erupted daily.*

I refused to maintain my weight when I left the hospital. My parents and doctors grew more anxious as I refused to comply with any rules. To my chagrin, a teacher was appointed to eat lunch with me every day. I was not allowed to teach swimming. My mom had to know exactly where I was at all times. As I lost more weight, further restrictions were placed on me.

I started seeing a psychiatrist, but I refused to "open up" to her. I wasn't prepared to admit that I had to change. I blamed my parents for all of my problems since they were the ones enforcing all of the rules and restrictions on me. I could not see how the eating disorder was robbing me of my freedom. The more my parents limited my activities, the more belligerent I became. At the same time, I was tormented by the worry and pain I was inflicting on my parents.

I kept a journal throughout my experiences. That fall I wrote, "I think about food and calories all the time. The worst part of it all is the look of sadness and disappointment on mom's face. Everything else I can handle." Soon thereafter I wrote, "I hate my life. I hate how I make everyone in my family frustrated and angry. I know I'm hurting everyone and that hurts me too, but I just can't help it. I am so selfish and miserable."

I wasn't prepared to admit that I had to change. I blamed my parents for all of my problems since they were the ones enforcing all of the rules and restrictions on me.

My parents and I began going to a weekly psychoeducation group run by the eating disorder program at our children's hospital. The goal of these sessions was to educate the group of parents and adolescents about eating disorders. In addition, the parents benefited from the moral support they got from each other and the group leaders. My "co-anorexics" and I used the time to compare "anorexia tricks" and to commiserate about how unfair we perceived our parents to be. After all, we were all angry that our parents were trying to sabotage our weight-loss strategies and trying to make us well.

All of our parents wondered the same thing — how did their sweet daughters become so angry and defiant before their eyes? It was particularly confusing since all of our parents were just following the doctor's orders and trying to help their daughters. An underlying frustration permeated the group. Parents are supposed to feed and nurture their children! What are parents supposed to do if their child refuses to be fed or nurtured? All the parents were scared of this powerful and potentially lethal illness that was threatening their daughters' lives.

Growing more independent and defiant...

Over the next few months, I refused to see things from my parents' perspective. The more incentives offered to me, the more I pulled away and focused on losing weight. I started seeing another child psychiatrist whom my parents and I liked a lot. However, even she could not pull me out from my starving abyss. I had no interest in getting better. I was more entrenched than ever before.

I also realized that when I turned 18 years old, my eating disorder team at the children's hospital would no longer have control over me. While I relished that thought, my parents were dreading the thought of having to cope with me without adequate support.

Three months before my 18th birthday, I was admitted to the hospital as a last resort. I was angry that I was being forced to gain weight against my will. I became even more determined to put up a fight. I had numerous admissions over that three-month period precipitated by a vicious cycle of weight fluctuations and defiant behavior. I was repeatedly admitted to the hospital against my will, gained weight even though I did my best to avoid eating, made empty promises involving meal plans and weight gain, and continued to beg my parents to discharge me. Out of physical and mental exhaustion, my parents would take me home. They knew that the hospitalizations were not helping me psychologically but were relieved that I was physically safe there.

I was repeatedly admitted to the hospital against my will, gained weight even though I did my best to avoid eating, made empty promises involving meal plans and weight gain, and continued to beg my parents to discharge me.

Outside the hospital, I was barely eating anything in an effort to compensate for the weight that I had been forced to gain as an inpatient. Our house was a battleground. When I was around, there was never any peace. My parents and three sisters suffered from my eating disorder, too. My parents were busy trying to cope with my eating disorder and me. This took away from their time and energy with the other girls. It was disruptive to our family's life to have me in and out of the hospital. When I was in the hospital, everyone talked about me, visited me, and anticipated me coming home. When I was home, everyone walked on eggshells. Everyone was frustrated and resentful. There was no normality in our lives.

Later that winter, I felt that my life had become a nightmare. I felt that my brain was holding me prisoner and I couldn't rationally sort out my thoughts. I was confused — I felt like a caged animal in the hospital, but the world outside the hospital was a scary, unpredictable place. My only escape from growing up was being in the hospital, where no one expected very much from me. I had an identity in the hospital. If I got well and moved on, I might lose this identity. I did not want to be forgotten by the hospital staff at the children's hospital.

I tried to make sense of my thoughts in my journal, "I am so afraid to turn 18 — no more security at the hospital. I don't ever want to go to into the adult eating disorder system. I kind of want to be in the hospital again. It is just so safe there and you get to eat always. I know it isn't reality but it is so secure. Also I can't deal with the weight gain. If I want to see my psychiatrist, I have to stay out. Moreover, I wanted to see her because in her presence everything feels good. But, I could run away from my problems temporarily in the hospital. I am so afraid to get better."

Every morning while I was in the hospital, I made my mom's life hell. After being weighed, I would be overwhelmed with anxiety. I would call her on the telephone screaming. She would try to calm me down, unsuccessfully. Over and over, she would hang up the telephone and I would call her back. The nurse would have to intervene and end this game. All day, I would provoke the staff by refusing my food. I would start arguments when I lost my privileges. I was so frustrated when all of my screams fell on deaf ears. My constant outbursts upset the other patients and disrupted the entire ward. My parents grew tired of hearing the reports about my latest antics.

When my mom came to visit, I would yell at her and intimidate her to take me home. On one specific occasion, my mom refused to take me home even after I begged and pleaded with her. She believed that I was not ready to go home and was not prepared to give in. In anger, I took her by the shoulders and shook her. My mom stared at me in shock and disbelief, her eyes welled with tears and she said, "You aren't my daughter. My daughter Tammy wouldn't act that

way. You are the anorexic monster inside of her who is trying
to take over."

In a way, she was right. It was almost as if I was possessed
by a horrible demon. I stopped caring about school, my family and friends. The only thing I cared about was being the
thinnest anorexic on the ward. But my parents, psychiatrist,
and the staff at the hospital were standing in my way. My
whole day would be consumed with thinking of ways to
avoid weight gain. I was so devious! I refused to take responsibility for hiding food or exercising,
despite the fact that the staff and patients
chastised and punished me for my behavior. As far as I was concerned, it wasn't
fair that I was in the hospital in the first
place. I told everyone that I was not sick
enough to be there and that my parents
were neglecting me by leaving me there.
My parents got the brunt of my anger. I
knew they loved me unconditionally and
would always forgive me, no matter how awful I behaved.

My mom stared at me in shock and disbelief, her eyes welled with tears and she said, "You aren't my daughter. My daughter Tammy wouldn't act that way.

At one point in the spring, the hospital staff felt they
could no longer meet my needs and they 'kicked me out' of
the hospital. My mother was not prepared to have me at
home and she did her best to watch me eat. After 2 days of
hiding food and constant arguments, she felt I had over-
stepped my boundaries. In utter frustration, she 'kicked me
out' of our home. She later felt badly and begged me to come
home. I refused to come back until she promised that she
would not watch me eat. When she agreed to get off my back,
I relented and came home. I felt I had won that battle, until I
was re-admitted to the hospital the following week. I felt so
lost and alone.

The thoughts going through my head caused me such anxiety and despair. I wrote in my journal, "I am pretty miserable
lately. I am all mixed up in the head and I don't know what to
do anymore. When I was home, I kept feeling like I wanted to
get better. But then, as it was time to eat, I panicked. I threw
stuff out right, left, and center. I never knew I was so devious
until this last weekend. What have I become?"

During my last admission at the children's hospital, I
made a conscious decision that as soon as I turned 18, I
would lose an excessive amount of weight. I convinced
myself that it would be my revenge — I wanted to get back
at the doctors and my parents for not allowing me to be thin

enough...ever. I convinced myself that once I achieved this extremely low weight, I would be ready to get better. I told my parents my plan and they pleaded with the doctors to help me. The plan made no sense to my parents. However, my pending 18th birthday symbolized my transformation to an adult, capable of making rational decisions. No one could do anything to stop me. While I was looking forward to breaking my ties with the children's hospital, I was secretly terrified of life in the adult world. I saw my friends graduating from high school and moving on. I felt unprepared to embark on the same journey. On the outside I appeared tough. On the inside, I was crying for help.

The week before my 18th birthday, I went on a tour of the adult eating disorder program. I made it clear to the program staff at the adult hospital, my parents, and my eating disorder team at the children's hospital that I had *no* interest in getting better. I still wanted to lose weight and punish everyone for forcing me to eat. I also wanted to hurt my parents for what I felt was their cruel behavior.

In a lucid moment...

After being discharged from my final hospitalization at the children's hospital, I spent the next 2 months losing weight. Instead of feeling free and happy, I was miserable. There was no glamor in a life of starvation. I missed the end of high school, ruined my summer, and upset everyone around me. I was sad, lonely, listless, and weak. No number on the scale was ever low enough. Every time I went to the doctor and got weighed, I felt the need to lose more weight. My biggest competition was other people with anorexia nervosa, whom I perceived as thinner and somehow more accomplished than me. Irrational thoughts governed my life. In a lucid moment, I came to an important realization. While I wanted the doctors to suffer, I was the real person who was suffering. It was time to find the strength within me to recover for my own self-worth and quality of life. The long and hard journey continued.

Whenever I would let my guard down, the "anorexic monster" reared its angry head. I learned the hard way that recovery had to be my top priority.

Ultimately, I went back to the adult eating disorder program to give it my best shot. With the dreadful memories of my previous summer still fresh in my mind, I used all of my energy to get well. I completed the adult program and tried to get involved in life. Unfortunately, I had a number of relapses and hospitalizations over the next few years. Whenever I would let my guard down, the "anorexic monster" reared its angry head. I learned the hard way that recovery had to be my top priority. As soon as I would give myself permission to lose a little weight, I would lose control over my symptoms and find myself in the midst of a relapse.

After my final discharge from the adult eating disorder program, I faced the sad reality that I had no life to go back to. My psychiatrist was on maternity leave. I felt I was destined to be sick forever. All that was familiar to me was "the illness." My future looked bleak. Until that point, I had never maintained a normal weight for longer than a few months before a relapse. My family was sick of the vicious cycle of watching me attempt recovery, relapse, and then end up in treatment again. They struggled with the possibility that I might never get better. My mom cried at the thought that I might never marry, go to school, or move on with my life. While I told my family that this time things would be different, they had their doubts. My mother said the same thing she had said every other time I had promised recovery, "Action speaks louder than words." Rather than speak about being ready to get well, I had to show myself and everyone else that I was serious about recovery.

Emerging from under a thick fog...

My mom gave me an ultimatum — demonstrate a true effort at getting well or find a new place to live. With that threat as a motivator, I felt as if I was emerging from under a thick fog. For the first time, I was able to acknowledge that my parents were looking out for my best interests by encouraging me to get well. I was not alone. I had friends and family who were willing to support me and help me...but no one could put the food in my mouth. I recognized that my "anorexic thoughts and behaviors" were alienating me from everyone around me. I came to terms with the fact that the "anorexic thoughts and behaviors" were the enemy! I had to use all of my artillery to fight them. Psychologically, I had reached rock bottom. I was ready to challenge my distorted thoughts and take responsibility for my recovery.

I believe that one factor that initially contributed to my recovery had to do with timing. When I left the hospital that summer, I had reached *my* time for getting well. Before that time, I was not ready to get well. There was no amount of external force that could work to help get me well.

The day of my discharge, I ate 'normally' outside of a hospital for the first time in years. To everyone's surprise, I continued eating, and my mother's ultimatum was forgotten. Even though the unknown of recovery was terrifying, I reminded myself that there had to be more to life than the misery that came with starving oneself. When I was ill, I wouldn't have believed it myself. Whenever a recovered patient tried to speak to me, I was never in the right headspace to listen. I wanted to give recovery a chance and I made eating an experiment — I had to try to eat on my own, and if it was horrible, I could always go back to my symptoms. But as time went on, I focused on getting involved with life to the point that I had no 'time' to relapse. I went back to school and avoided socializing with unhealthy individuals. With the help of my doctor and therapist, I stopped playing the starvation game and I experimented with living. Instead of waiting for my negative thoughts to change before eating, I put the food in my mouth regardless of my irrational thoughts. To my surprise, the 'anorexic thoughts' got quieter and eating and gaining weight became easier.

The long journey...

My family and I have traveled over a long journey since that August 7 years ago. Since that fateful summer, we have endured many challenging experiences. I am now 24 years old and an active participant in life. I am in graduate school. I have a good family and great friends who supported me through this difficult journey. I couldn't have made it this far without them. As well, I am forever grateful to my doctors and psychiatrists who never gave up on me, no matter how difficult I was.

I volunteer and help those less fortunate. I have an appreciation for life that many others don't have. I have a desire to live. I know I am a person with worth, and it has nothing to do with a number on a scale. I am focused on my future.

So, that is my story. I know that there are many young people who struggle with many of the same issues that I have struggled with. Many have recovered. I used to think that starving myself made me unique and special. As I met more patients with eating disorders, I realized how we were all the same...we all had tricks, we knew how to lose weight, and we were all champions at self-destruction. When I was starving, I was not different than the other young people with anorexia nervosa who were starving themselves.

As I embraced recovery, I came to terms with the fact that I am more unique when I eat and develop my character. I am a unique daughter, friend, and individual. While my negative thoughts haven't gone away completely, winning the battle means eating despite the self-sabotaging thoughts. I can transcend and come out victorious, and I hope your child can too.

I still have my struggles. I regard my recovery as quite an accomplishment for someone who thought life outside the hospital was impossible. Like most people, I face new challenges every day. However, I have learned to cope with these challenges in a more constructive way. Recovery isn't an all-or-nothing experience — for me it is somewhere in between. I am quite comfortable with where I am today. I have been through many treatment programs and have done a lot of soul-searching. The more I experience and learn, the more I realize that I have self-worth.

Like most people, I face new challenges every day. However, I have learned to cope with these challenges in a more constructive way. Recovery isn't an all-or-nothing experience — for me it is somewhere in between.

I used to be obsessed with the fact that I had never been the 'sickest' or the 'thinnest' anorexic. Now, as I am able to focus on what is truly important in life, I no longer *want* to be known as the sickest. I am motivated to build a healthy identity where my life does not revolve around hospital admissions or doctors and nurses remembering me. I was just a patient to them — I want people in the 'real world' to acknowledge me and accept me for who I am. I have made new friends, and many of them don't know that I've been to hell and back. It's my own secret. I know where I've been and I am so proud of how hard I have worked to get where I am today.

No, it hasn't been easy or fun, but it is worthwhile. I have learned to focus my energy on health and wellness. Instead of trying to be the 'perfect anorexic,' I accept myself for who I am. I feel good about myself by helping others and doing my part to contribute to the world. The important thing is, I have started to like myself and have decided to get well *for me*; not for my parents or the doctors. Instead of hiding in hospital, I want to experience life for myself. My life today is so much more fulfilling than life with an active eating disorder ever was.

ADVICE FOR PARENTS

It is difficult for me to write to parents, since I have never been one. I wish I had answers to all the important and difficult questions about having an eating disorder and recovering from one…but I don't. I hope that through my story, you will understand a little bit more about what life is like for an adolescent with an eating disorder. Even though each of us is different, there are similarities between my experience and others who suffer from an eating disorder. I have gained a tremendous amount of insight over the years and have some advice to share.

Eating Disorders Are Complex

I remember hearing people ask my parents why they never just "made me eat." Forcing a person to eat will not make him or her better — healing the psychological component to eating disorders is vital in the recovery process. As much as my parents would have liked to cure me, there were complex psychological issues that worked as a barrier.

Unfortunately, there is no quick fix or magic pill that can treat an eating disorder. Early on, my parents worked hard to force me into treatment so that I could get well. I understand now why they did this. They couldn't stand there and wait for me to change. It helped them to call doctors, go to groups, and look into treatment options. At the time, I was very angry with them for sabotaging my elaborate starvation plan. I used to yell and scream at them for hospitalizing me and make them feel guilty for not allowing me to starve. Parents are responsible for keeping their children healthy — no matter what reactions they get from their sick child.

Being Informed Is Vital

First, there are a lot of uninformed individuals who assume that people with eating disorders are starving themselves to get attention and to be skinny. This is not true. Eating disorders are serious mental illnesses that symbolize deeper issues within the individual.

When I was actively starving myself, I felt overwhelmed with life and the demands of adolescence. Instead of telling my parents, I starved myself to cope with my fears. It is important for parents and the public at large to understand that eating disorders are more than just a desire to be thin. There are always deeper issues at hand.

Eating Disorders Come in All Shapes, Weights, and Sizes

During my experience, I met a number of people who were normal weight or overweight and suffering from the debilitating psychological effects of an eating disorder. There is a misconception that if young people have an eating disorder, they have to look emaciated. Again, this is not true!

People with eating disorders may be at a normal weight or overweight. Being under the false impression that one needs to be 'skinny' to have an eating disorder often makes normal or overweight adolescents with eating disorders feel as if they are 'not really' sick enough and do not require help. People with an eating disorder, regardless if their weight, shape, or size, deserves to get the help they need in order to get better. Not everyone has to be 50 pounds before they 'deserve' treatment. Remember, eating disorders are about a frame of mind, not a number on a scale.

The Eating Disorder Is the Illness, Not the Person

When I was in the throes of my illness, I had the intense feeling that I couldn't survive if I ate more or gained weight. At the same time, I was ashamed and guilty about my problem and I was very hard on myself for being so difficult. My family worked incredibly hard to separate the *anorexia nervosa* from *me*, their child.

It was comforting to know that my parents were frustrated and angry with the *illness*, as opposed to being frustrated and angry with me. This helped me feel less responsible for being such a burden on everyone. Consequently, parents and siblings must try to recognize that most often the strong feelings are directed toward the *eating disorder* and not their sick adolescent.

Parents Don't Cause Eating Disorders

Many people are uninformed about the causes, severity, and treatment of eating disorders. Some people have the false impression that my parents were 'bad' and caused my anorexia nervosa. No, parents don't cause an eating disorder.

My parents felt a tremendous amount of guilt when I was first diagnosed with anorexia nervosa. They blamed themselves for letting me get sick. They constantly wondered whether they had caused my eating disorder. Parents need to know that medical research has shown that eating disorders are not caused by parents but are caused by a complex combination of factors.

I understand that my parents did not 'cause' my problems. In fact, I have stopped looking for the cause of my eating disorder. I realize that there is no point in searching for the cause. The focus should be the recovery and looking toward the future.

Parents Can Prevent Abnormal Eating Attitudes and Behaviors

While parents cannot directly cause their child's eating disorder, there are ways that parents can help prevent abnormal eating attitudes and behaviors. Parents should avoid criticizing their own bodies or discussing weight loss in front of their children. How can children accept their bodies if their own parents are unhappy with their own bodies?

In addition, families should not label foods as "good" or "bad." Families should avoid commenting on the type and quantity of food eaten by others. Children should be accepted at all shapes and sizes. Teenagers live in a world where they are bombarded with unrealistic images of skinny actresses and models. If parents can start at home to teach their children that self-worth is independent of weight and shape, we can enable teens to enjoy a healthy life.

Parents Can Support Their Child with an Eating Disorder

My mother was proactive and couldn't stand by and watch me destroy my life. She said that if I had been diagnosed with cancer, she would have searched the world for the best oncologists to get me better. Seeing me suffer and not being able to find the experts to find an immediate 'cure' left her feeling helpless and frustrated.

I no longer blame her for doing her best to help me. I understand that I might not be here today if she had given up on me.

Parents and Siblings Need to Take Care of Themselves

Parents and siblings of the sufferer have to take care of their own mental well-being as well. For my family, it meant attending support groups and seeing their own individual therapists. Having a loved one with a chronic mental illness takes a major toll on everyone involved.

It was important for my mom to speak to a therapist so that she could vent her frustration and anger. The therapist validated her feelings and frustrations and provided her with support. The therapist confirmed that my mom was doing the right thing in trying to help me. My mom had a lot of competing demands — she had to raise my sisters, keep her marriage together, and keep her sanity. She learned that she had to take care of herself in order to help our family. She could not allow herself to wallow in worry and self-blame.

Recovery Is a Hard and Long Process

Parents must come to terms with the fact that recovery from an eating disorder can take years. My family was under the false impression that I would recover from my eating disorder after one short hospital admission.

The long, hard, and rocky road to recovery is a very difficult concept to 'wrap your head around.' Parents find it completely illogical when their daughter or son starves themselves or binges and purges. At the same time it seems so logical to 'just eat' and 'get better.' Unfortunately, there is nothing rational about an eating disorder.

The recovery process is a combination of peaks and valleys. Families must be prepared to deal with a child who may be ambivalent, moody, angry, frightened, guilty, lacking in confidence, and very confused. There is no one model for recovery…every individual is different. Just as the disorder did not develop overnight, it won't go away overnight either.

PART 3

Family and Community Roles in Recovery and Prevention

CHAPTER 16

Everyone Needs Help

What happens to the family when they have a child or adolescent with an eating disorder? Yes, children with eating disorders suffer, but they are not alone. All family members suffer when there is a child with an eating disorder in the home. Parents, siblings, and the family as a whole are affected by the physical, emotional, and social consequences when a young person has an eating disorder. As one parent noted, "Anorexia engulfs not only the sufferer but also those who come in contact with it."

While eating disorders may disrupt the family, you, as a family, have the energy and resources to cope with the eating disorder. Your immediate and extended family can help your child return to a normal pattern of family life.

How Is Family Life Affected?

Very few normal family functions remain after living with an eating disordered person. The longer the eating disorder persists, the greater is the disruption to normal family functioning.

Family Routines

All families develop routines to handle regular responsibilities and expectations in family life. These routines provide an element of stability and predictability, guiding family members on how they will relate to each other. Taken together, these family patterns help define the members in a particular family and give a sense of family identity. Taking on the responsibility for the care and supervision of a child with an eating disorder will interrupt these routines.

Mealtimes

Most families take for granted that mealtime is a pleasurable activity that brings all the members of the family together in a shared experience. This is not the case when the family includes a child or adolescent with an eating disorder. Instead, mealtimes are transformed into a power struggle for control.

? Did You Know...

• Professionals who study family responses to illness use the term "caregiver distress" to describe the presence of problems and adverse events that affect individual family members and overall family functioning.

• Sometimes parents are so focused on the struggles of their ill child that they minimize the disruption to their own lives and those of other family members.

WORKSHEET

FAMILY CONSEQUENCES SCALE

A Family Consequences Scale can assist families in understanding the specific impact the eating disorder is having on them. Applying the results of this questionnaire is relatively simple. The higher the number of "Yes" answers, the greater the impact of the eating disorder on your family. This scale may be helpful in confirming the extent of the disruption to your family's life; strengthening your decision to act; and identifying problem areas requiring immediate attention.

Question	Yes	No
Do you feel guilty or blame yourself for your child's eating disorder?	☐	☐
Have you changed mealtimes?	☐	☐
Have mealtimes become an emotional battleground between you and your child?	☐	☐
Do you invite people to visit your home less frequently?	☐	☐
Do you find yourself looking for excuses not to attend social events within the extended family?	☐	☐
Are you afraid to go out and leave your child unattended?	☐	☐
Have you made alterations to your kitchen or dining areas – e.g., installed locks on the refrigerator or cupboards, added a locked door?	☐	☐
Do you inspect your child's room on a regular basis?	☐	☐
Do you accompany your child to the bathroom or monitor it afterward for signs of purging?	☐	☐
Have you made deliberate changes to your parenting style?	☐	☐
Do you find it increasingly difficult to trust what your child says to you?	☐	☐
Have you tried to stop your child from exercising or set limits on the amount of exercise?	☐	☐
Are you tormented by worry or fear over the health of your child?	☐	☐
Have your own eating and sleeping patterns changed?	☐	☐
Do you feel physically and mentally exhausted?	☐	☐
Do you and your partner find yourself in more arguments and conflicts than in the past?	☐	☐
Has your ability to perform your job been negatively affected?	☐	☐
Are you able to give your other children the attention they need?	☐	☐
Have the relationships between your son or daughter and their siblings been adversely affected by the eating disorder?	☐	☐
Does it feel like the eating disorder has come to occupy the central place in your family's life?	☐	☐

Watching a child deliberately starve compels parents to change the regular routine if it will encourage eating. Parents will change the time or location of the meal, prepare different foods for different family members, and even abandon the expectation that the whole family will eat together. Unfortunately, most of these changes fail to achieve the desired result.

These behaviors upset the family meal routine. While parents may be frustrated or worried, siblings may feel angry with their sister or brother for not eating normally and changing the previously enjoyable course of family mealtime.

Q: **My daughter has anorexia nervosa and must eat three meals and three snacks a day. Every time we sit down to a meal, it's a struggle. What can we do?**

A: Start by accepting that struggles will be part of mealtime for a considerable period of time and prepare yourself emotionally for the challenges that lay ahead. Knowing in advance what to expect will help minimize some of the negative feelings that you may experience. Understanding that the emotional onslaught is part of the disorder will help you not to take things personally and prevent you from blaming your child.

In addition, you can be proactive in finding ways to support yourself after meals. This may involve taking the time to speak with your partner, treating yourself to quiet time with a book, going for a walk, or talking on the phone with a friend. What you do is less important than actually doing something that allows you to manage the stress of mealtime.

Social Isolation

The sharing of food is an integral part of most social occasions. Parents of a child with an eating disorder often find themselves in a difficult position socially as they try to avoid public conflict with their child, hide their child's physical condition, and spare themselves unwanted criticism.

Parents may isolate their family from their relatives, friends, neighbors, and acquaintances. This occurs slowly over time, until one day, parents suddenly realize that isolation and secrecy have become a part of their new lifestyle. This unintended consequence results in parents being cut off from important sources of personal support that might help them to deal more effectively with their child's eating disorder.

Focus of Attention

Many families find that the eating disorder and the teen with the eating disorder become the exclusive focus of attention, influencing almost all parts of family life. Changes to family routines are not only inconvenient, but leave family members feeling uncomfortable, lost, and disoriented. Individual family members often ask, "What happened to the family that I used to know?"

Family Roles

Eating disorders require parents to change how they interact with their child who is ill. Often this means taking on a whole new role.

Food Police

One of the first and most difficult of these new roles is that parents find themselves functioning as the 'food police'. Parents may assume this role when they try to intervene to ensure that their son or daughter maintains their health.

In families where the child struggles with anorexia nervosa, the parents may set menu plans, impose consequences for not eating, and limit exercise. In families where the child struggles with bulimia nervosa, the parents may need to limit access to food, limit the time in the bathroom after meals, and put locks on the refrigerator or kitchen cabinet doors. This policing role is uncomfortable for the parents, the child, and the immediate family. It can trigger prolonged conflict and animosity.

Hands-On Parenting

In response to their child's eating disorder, mothers and fathers are often forced to modify their age-appropriate approach to parenting. Adolescence is a time of significant physical, emotional, and intellectual changes as teenagers make the transition to adulthood. In order for parents to let go and allow their children to become more independent, they have to trust that their son or daughter will make responsible decisions that do not put themselves at risk. This normal developmental task is disrupted by an eating disorder and may require the parent to intercede assertively.

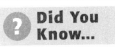

Did You Know...

● Children with eating disorders may actually regress physically, psychologically, and emotionally.

● Parents may need to take a more 'hands-on' approach consistent with parenting younger children.

Relationships

Personal relationships are the emotional bonds that hold families together. Eating disorders disrupt the well-being of the whole family by attacking these emotional connections among family members.

Parent-Child Relationships

The first relationship to suffer is the parents' relationship with their child. Changes in this relationship may start before you become aware of the eating disorder, as your child becomes gradually distanced from family life. As the eating disorder progresses in its severity, parents become alarmed by the startling transformation in their child's personality. Their previously quiet, compliant, and respectful son or daughter appears to have been replaced by a willful, stubborn, and angry child who rejects all parental contact and influence.

The painful situation described by this mother is typical. "Ruth has become an ungrateful, rude, manipulative, and totally self-controlled individual who is subject to violent mood swings. She has always been a quiet introverted individual who worries about everything but is very low...this change has been very difficult for us to come to terms with." It is no wonder that many parents are left sadly shaking their heads and asking themselves, "Who is this stranger who has come into our lives?"

Couple Relationships

An adolescent with an eating disorder can place unbearable pressure on the parents' spousal relationship. Having to change family routines and cope with unrelenting emotional stress can lead to several predictable outcomes. First, even in healthy marriages, partners may experience more conflict with each other in the presence of a child with an eating disorder. These new tensions can increase existing disagreements within the marriage. Conflicts can also arise about equal sharing of the responsibility for the care of the ill child. Finally, there may be differences in opinion on how best to manage the situation.

Sibling Relationships

Sibling relationships are also affected by an adolescent's eating disorder. Powerful and conflicting emotions are stirred up in the other children. This can temporarily weaken the sibling's relationship with the affected teen.

Family Authority

In most families, relationships are organized with parents serving as the family executive, making decisions for the well-being and safety of their children. This traditional authority is altered in families where an adolescent has an eating disorder. The threat of not eating is so powerful that it can allow the child with the eating disorder to dictate to parents. As a result, intelligent and caring parents will find themselves giving in, contrary to sound decisions they had previously made.

CASE STUDY Susan

Susan's mother had a private fantasy. "What would it be like to be single again? Working full-time? Having a life of my own?" She loved her job, but had gone part-time when Susan was diagnosed with the eating disorder. She also thought about what it would be like to take the other kids and leave Susan with her dad. They were 'two peas from the same pod' in many ways. Being a single mother of four seemed easy compared to taking care of Susan and coping with her dad. What happened to the man she had fallen in love with. When had he turned into such an angry man?

As she was thinking about this, she got a call on her cell phone. It was her husband, yelling and screaming about how she had forgotten to pick up his dry cleaning. Something in her snapped! After all she had given up, including her job, it came down to his dry cleaning. She had had enough. She told him that, from now on, he was responsible for the dry cleaning and *his*

daughter. She quit! She was giving up her job as Susan's mother and as his servant. There was silence on the other end. "Are you leaving me?" he asked. "I don't know," she answered. She hung up and drove home.

When she got home, it was just the two of them — husband and wife. The kids were gone. He had sent them to his mother's place for a sleepover. They were alone. She couldn't remember the last time this had happened. It didn't take long before the two of them were in tears. They talked for hours about the toll Susan's eating disorder had taken on them individually, as a couple, and as a family.

They decided that they needed to talk to a professional about their marital relationship and the family relationships. They decided to go for marital therapy. As a family who had not believed in this head-shrinking business, they were now the most 'therapized' couple on the block.

continued on page 265

Emotional Turmoil

An eating disorder unleashes an emotional earthquake within the family, taking a terrible toll on everyone. Eating disorders can leave parents feeling defeated and demoralized, siblings confused and resentful.

Escalating Conflicts

Parents and children can find themselves locked into destructive, repetitive interactions with a predictable set of outcomes.

In one scenario, the child lashes out verbally at the parents with such hateful fury that the parents eventually stop demanding their child to eat. In another situation, the adolescent shuts down completely — both verbally and emotionally — and the parents watch helplessly. The final scenario is one where the child uses the threat of not eating anything to win parental agreement for eating small amounts of food.

A distraught father describes this last situation as follows: "We were scared to death of her not eating. We were walking on eggshells because the smallest upset made her threaten not to eat even the little she had agreed to."

Denial and Defiance

In addition to mealtimes, there are a number of other situations that regularly lead to conflict. To begin, adolescents with eating disorders frequently deny anything is wrong and reject offers of help. When a parent tries to manage the symptoms of the eating disorder or arrange treatment, their child responds with hostility, resistance, or verbal assault.

Guilt, Anger, and Fear

Most parents find themselves affected by a range of powerful feelings. They may feel guilty that this situation is somehow their fault. They may feel helpless in not being able to stop their daughter or son from starving themselves. Parents may feel ashamed that they have failed in their role as caregivers, grief for the loss of the previous relationship with their child, and pain from the verbal abuse that is directed their way.

Parents may experience anger at the difficulties they encounter in seeking treatment; disgust at having to clean up after a binge or purging episode; and profound sadness over the changes that have occurred in their family life. Parents may be terrified that their child could die from this unrelenting disorder.

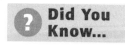

Did You Know...

• Young people with eating disorders will often respond negatively to their parents' attempts to limit access to food in the home and to reduce freedoms and privileges previously enjoyed.

• Over time, this pattern of conflict becomes ingrained and the whole emotional climate of the family changes.

IN THEIR OWN WORDS

Parents who have supported their child through this stressful experience have a great deal of hard-earned knowledge and wisdom to share. Hearing how their families have been affected by their child's eating disorder may help you in coping with the impact on your family. These comments have been excerpted from various studies of a parent's experience of caring for a child with an eating disorder.

- "When someone is screaming at you and swearing at you because she is hungry and tired and malnourished, it's really hard to take a step back and be objective. Every time we had a meal, we felt that we were verbally assaulted."

- "The mother of an anorexic has the bitter experience of having her love and nurturing, symbolically herself, rejected."

- "A doleful procession of adverse events, a crescendo of anxiety and woe that was hard for us to handle."

- "I find it difficult to talk about Hannah's illness with people, partly because I feel like I'm a failure if I need to share my worries or ask for help and partly because of the few friends I have confided in, only one has offered any real support, while the others have distanced themselves."

- "As a mother, you hope your children will gradually become more independent, but the reverse seems to be the case. We seem to be going backwards."

- "Professionals were secretive and we felt patronized. Everyone seemed to feel that we were 'bad parents' because our child had anorexia nervosa, and this made it all the harder for our family."

Physical and Mental Health Consequences

Having a child with an eating disorder in the family unit can have serious health and behavior consequences for the parents and the siblings.

Parents

Even the strongest parents are worn down by the challenges of living with a child suffering from an eating disorder. It is not surprising that some parents experience physical and mental health problems. Some parents may experience a change in appetite, difficulties sleeping, increasing social isolation, new physical problems (headaches, stomach problems), and new emotional difficulties (anxiety and depression). Parents need to take care of themselves so that they are better able to care for their child with an eating disorder.

Problems at Work

The added effects of managing a child's eating disorder may eventually create problems at a parent's workplace. Realistically, going to the numerous doctor and therapy appointments, being available if your child is hospitalized, and supporting your child in any way possible will take time away from the workplace. A parent's ability to concentrate in the workplace can also be undermined by constant worry.

In households where both parents work outside the home, it may be necessary for one or both to re-negotiate the terms of their employment to make more time available. This may have consequences for career advancement and the family's financial situation.

Frustrations with Health-Care Professionals

Some parents report difficult interactions with health-care professionals as they seek help for their child's eating disorder. Some families struggle to be heard and to be taken seriously when they seek help. Apparently careless comments, such as "Take him home and feed him a hamburger" or "It's just a phase she's going through," only add to the burden of confusion and pain that parents experience. Depending on the philosophy of the treatment center, parents may feel they are either blamed as the cause of the eating disorder, or, alternatively, they are not treated as an integral part of the treatment team.

Unfortunately, for some parents, the pain and confusion does not stop when their child enters treatment. Frequently, health-care professionals fail to prepare parents for the realities of treatment. If the health-care professionals fail to lay the groundwork for the course of this tenacious illness, it can ultimately undermine the treatment and threaten the relationship among the treatment team, the parents, and the child.

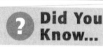

? Did You Know...

• If parents are to support their child with an eating disorder, they may need to get professional help for themselves, individually or as a couple.

• Think about joining parent support or psychoeducational groups. Learning from others who have experienced a similar situation can be quite helpful.

CASE STUDY Martha

Martha's brother asked his parents if he could move out and live at his uncle's. Martha's parents were shocked. Why would he want to leave them? He told them that he was tired of living with a "crazy person." Martha's eating disorder was ruining his life.

His parents were puzzled. Martha had been doing better lately. Why now? "Well," he said, "it's only a matter of time before something new happens…if it's not purging, it's stealing, and if it's not stealing then what…drugs?" His parents immediately asked him if he knew something he wasn't telling them. "Was Martha doing drugs?"

"No!" he yelled. "But of course it always comes back to Martha — you've already forgotten that I'm leaving. This is why I am leaving."

Martha's parents realized that he was right. In fact, when they talked to all the boys, they realized just how bad things were. The boys realized that Martha was taking up so much of their parent's time and energy, they couldn't possibly ask their parents for anything. All the boys felt like they needed to be on their best behavior. They did their schoolwork and household chores without being asked. They tried not to cause their parents any problems. But it was getting hard for all of them to be good boys, good sons, and good brothers. Martha's parents decided that things would have to change and that no one would be leaving.

continued on page 259

Siblings

Children with eating disorder require a great deal of attention. As a result, their siblings often feel neglected and abandoned.

Uncertainty and Confusion

Siblings also find themselves caught up in an emotional roller coaster when they have a sister or brother with an eating disorder. Initially, siblings have feelings of anxiety and concern for the adolescent with an eating disorder. However, as the eating disorder intensifies, the sibling may withdraw this initial support or become more confused.

As conflict in the household increases and routines change or disappear, brothers or sisters often become increasingly frustrated with the sibling who is ill. Their changing feelings go from concern to confusion to anger, and then to a sense of uncertainty and guilt. They think, "How can I be angry at my brother or sister whose life is threatened by this illness?" Brothers and sisters feel an emotional turmoil very similar to that of their parents.

HELP FOR YOUR FAMILY

Parents can do a great deal to help all family members cope with the eating disorder and help the child with the eating disorder on the road to recovery. Consider the following suggestions.

☐ **Take Stock of Your Family's Situation**

Living with a child who has an eating disorder makes it difficult for parents 'to see the forest for the trees' when it comes to appreciating the toll on the family. Questionnaires like the Family Consequences Scale may be helpful in identifying the extent to which individual lives and family interactions have been affected.

☐ **Seek Accurate Information**

Eating disorders are complex mental health problems that are not easily understood by the community at large, by family members affected by a child with the disorder, or by some health-care professionals. If you have been struggling on your own with limited family or professional support, it is important that you locate specialized eating disorder resources that can help you better understand what you and your child are up against.

☐ **Support the Siblings**

Parents and health-care providers need to be sensitive to the unique needs of siblings. You can help your other children learn more about eating disorders and discuss how these disorders directly and indirectly have an impact on their lives. Siblings should feel free to express their questions and concerns. Parents and health-care professionals need to be aware of the sibling's understanding of the disorder, their adjustment, and their behavior.

☐ **Get Back to Family Basics**

Even though you have a child suffering with an eating disorder, make an effort to re-establish as many traditional family routines as possible. Returning to the old and familiar ways will increase the emotional comfort of family members. Ultimately, it will help the family to feel less 'stuck' in a difficult problem that seems beyond solution.

☐ **Work Together as Parents**

Research studies have shown that parental mood and adjustment to a child's chronic illness will have an impact on their children's ability to cope with the situation. Both parents need to be working together to develop a shared approach on how to deal with the situation. One of the most important components of a successful outcome for a child with an eating disorder is when both parents provide a unified approach to treatment. Talk to each other. Work together for your child.

☐ **Ask for Professional Help**

Keep in mind that members of your family may need professional help. Skilled eating disorder specialists can help you and your family members reduce conflict, support each other more effectively, and restore some balance in the family.

Sense of Loss

Siblings often experience a sense of loss for the relationship they had with their brother or sister before they became ill. "Sometimes I am struck by a picture of my brother aged 10," a young family member once remarked, "one with all rosy cheeks and smiles, up to no good and full of energy. At these times, I indulge myself in thinking of what he could be now if he was not anorexic. I grieve for the brother I think I have lost."

Siblings can experience another sense of loss. The parents' preoccupation with the child with an eating disorder means less time and energy for the other children. If the needs of the siblings are not adequately met, it can potentially affect their emotional health and development.

Extra Effort

Some siblings of children with eating disorders appear to go out of their way to take on extra tasks and be supportive in the family. They may also avoid bringing personal issues to their parents. Whether these siblings are acting on their own initiative or whether they are responding to direct or indirect messages that the family is overburdened is not clear. This increased sense responsibility may be expressed in caring for younger children in the household when parents are busy with the needs of the child with the eating disorder.

> **? Did You Know…**
>
> ● Siblings of children with eating disorders should not be expected to take on adult responsibilities.
>
> ● Research studies have shown that this increase in responsibility, coupled with a decrease in parental attention, can lead to anxiety, depression, and poor psychological development in the siblings.

Q: My daughter was diagnosed with an eating disorder six months ago. Since then, there is no time left for our younger son. What should we do?

A: You have to make time for your son. Split or share the responsibility with your partner. Rather than both of you going to appointments with your daughter, one can accompany your daughter while the other spends time with your son. Time spent with your son will not only be a welcome opportunity to enjoy this relationship, but it will provide a respite from the stressful duties of caring for a child with an eating disorder.

CHAPTER 17

Helping Yourself to Help Your Child

When a child has been diagnosed with an eating disorder, parents typically ask themselves, "Where did we go wrong? What did we do to contribute to this?" Parents often feel that they must have made some horrible mistake for this to happen to their child. This unrelenting feeling of guilt is generally unavoidable, but parents need to understand there is no evidence that parents cause their child's eating disorder.

Rather than feeling guilty about something in the past, parents should be asking, "What can I do now to support my child and family through this challenging task of treating this eating disorder?" To help your child and family, though, you may need support from your relatives, friends, and community, as well as the health-care team treating your child.

Parents also need to take care of themselves. Having a child with an eating disorder can be exhausting. It may feel as though you have no time for yourself or for other members of your family. If you don't make time for yourself, all family members, including your child with the eating disorder, may suffer.

If you have ever flown on a plane, you will remember the opening announcements of the cabin crew regarding what to do in the case of an emergency. They always emphasize the need for those traveling with children to bring the oxygen mask to their own mouth before assisting the child. The reason for this is that adults will not be able to help their children if they do not help themselves first.

This analogy is true for many situations, including parenting your child through their struggle with an eating disorder. You will only be able to help your child if you are looking after yourself as well. This may include taking some time off work, calling on friends and family members to help with such tasks as driving and child care, delegating responsibilities that formerly only you could do, and, of course, getting enough sleep and eating in a healthy way. Take a walk, call a friend, or find some quiet time for yourself.

? Did You Know...

• If asking for help does not come easily to you, finding support may be a challenge. Many children with eating disorders also find it very difficult to ask for help.

• For your daughter or son to see you reaching out for assistance may encourage them to follow suit. Your positive role modeling has the potential to be more helpful than any form of therapy.

Q: Sometimes I feel like I'm to blame for my child's eating disorder. What did I do wrong as a parent?

A: There is no evidence to suggest that any specific style of parenting or characteristic of a parent causes an eating disorder. If you are experiencing guilt or negative feelings about your ability to parent your child, try to talk to someone you trust. Blaming yourself could increase any lack of confidence you may be experiencing around your parenting skills.

You are going to need a great deal of confidence in yourself to take on your child's eating disorder symptoms. Requiring your daughter or son to do things that they do not want to do will take strength and courage; this will elude you if you are blaming yourself. If you become stuck with negative thoughts about your abilities and self-blame about your child's illness, you will be less able to help your child to become 'unstuck'.

Sources of Support

In your effort to support your child, you may find valuable support from health-care professionals, support groups, your extended family, and friends. Other forms of support, such as family therapy and psychoeducation groups, are also valuable for keeping your family informed, involved, and together as a unit.

Professional Support

Support for yourself may include speaking to a counselor or therapist on your own. This may involve one session or multiple sessions throughout the duration of your child's illness. For some people, counseling or therapy may seem like a foreign or unfamiliar course of action. But as you become more familiar with your child's treatment team, it may become easier to discuss this option with them, or you may discuss this with someone outside the treatment team — your family doctor or pediatrician, for example, or an employee assistance counselor at work.

Support Groups

Family members who have a teen with an eating disorder are often in need of a supportive environment. Many communities offer support groups, either through mental-health agencies or through local eating disorder programs or coalitions. Support groups range in type and format. Groups may be open or closed.

In an open group, people can join at any time and leave at any time. A wide range of people tend to be involved in these ongoing groups, which can be beneficial. A closed group generally has a fixed start and end date and a set number of sessions. The group is usually closed to new members after the second or third week of sessions, allowing for the added benefit of creating a group where members can come to feel they know the others well, with a strong sense of group cohesion.

Some groups are supportive in nature, exploring how the experience of coping with an eating disorder has been for family members. Other groups may have a more structured style, such as psychoeducation groups (groups that provide education about eating disorders) or skills-based groups.

Groups will also vary in terms of which family members attend. Some groups are parent-only groups, some are for parents and teens with eating disorders, while others are for parents and siblings of the child with the eating disorder.

Choice of groups may be limited to what is offered in your community. If you have a range of options, try to find a format that fits you.

Q: We are very private people. We do not want to talk about our family life with strangers. What is so valuable about family group therapy?

A: For families who have children with eating disorders, the American Academy of Psychiatry states that family therapy should be considered whenever possible. You should consider discussing any hesitancy you may have about family therapy with the social worker or psychiatrist working with your child. You may want to start with a parent-only meeting or attend a family psychoeducation group. Your ideas about what makes sense for your family may change over time, and the best time to begin family therapy may vary between families. Family counseling is often a good opportunity for brothers and sisters to express their concerns and be assisted in knowing what they should do.

ADVICE FROM OTHER PARENTS

Parents of children with eating disorders have found that one of the most powerful forms of support is speaking with other parents who have experienced or are experiencing a similar situation. You may find support and comfort in these words of advice for parents from other parents with children who have eating disorders.

"Remember your family strengths and continue to show appreciation for each other."

"Protect 'time off' from the problem. Make sure you spend time with other family members. Make sure you protect some time for yourself."

"Develop a clear plan that you review with others who have responsibility and are directly involved with your child's physical and mental health."

"Do not get involved in continuous negotiations and re-negotiations with your child about how much needs to be eaten, when it needs to be eaten, and how quickly it needs to be eaten. If a discussion is going nowhere, take a break. If a pattern of making compromises around eating disorder attitudes and behaviors is well established, it will be difficult to reverse."

"Don't give responsibility to younger or older brothers and sisters to take care of your child's eating disorder behaviors. They may be asked to monitor what their sister eats or scold her when she doesn't eat. This is not a role for a sibling to take on. Siblings often report that they get very little direction from parents or the treatment team about what to do and how to cope. This type of interaction between siblings is generally not well received by the child with the eating disorder.

Should We Change Our Parenting Style?

Caring for a child with an eating disorder often results in parents questioning their own parenting style. These questions can be very upsetting. For parents who have historically been confident about how to parent their children, it can be very disconcerting to feel defeated and rejected no matter what they do or say.

Once the presence of an eating disorder is acknowledged, parents generally find that it is helpful to review their parenting style and develop a united response to the eating disorder symptoms. Parents may need to change their style of parenting in part. Sometimes you can make these changes yourself; other times you may need support from family counselors.

Rules and Expectations

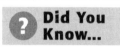

Did You Know...

• Your child may not be able to appreciate that your consistent and unrelenting involvement is an expression of commitment, love, and responsibility.

Parents should consider a set of rules and expectations that will be in place in their home so that the eating disorder does not control their child and take over their family life. Handling everyday eating disorder situations, such as refusal to eat, dieting, vomiting, overactivity, weight tampering, or laxative abuse, will be difficult. Strong emotions will be in place on both sides. Parents often report not knowing what to do.

Young people with eating disorders may reject the need for parental involvement in managing their eating disorder symptoms. They may state over and over, "I can do this on my own!" Parents may choose to back off if their previously loving, affectionate, compliant child accuses them of being mean, unfair, or punitive. Parents who have worked hard to provide a fair and democratic environment in their home may be insulted if their child refers to them as "strict."

Ordinary Teenage Behaviors

In addition to responding to the eating disorder symptoms, there may be other normal teenage behaviors that need a calm, firm, parental response. For example, your daughter or son might be rude, not participate in clean up, or not abide by the rules for the use of the car or curfews. Every parent will face one or all of these types of issues during the adolescent years.

However, the challenges of coping with a child who has an eating disorder should not be a license for you to tolerate unacceptable behavior. If you have other children, they will become confused if there are different rules for the child with an eating disorder as opposed to those who do not have an eating disorder.

Q: I'm becoming concerned about my other child's eating habits. What should I do?

A: Variations in eating habits of other family members can occur for a variety of reasons. Family members may feel more stressed or feel neglected due to the degree of concern for the child with an eating disorder. Having had one child diagnosed with an eating disorder can heighten a parent's sensitivity to what their other children are eating. Maintaining vigilance about meal times, menu planning, and keeping in tune with your other children may at times be more than you can manage. Speaking openly to your other children about your concerns would be a first step. If your concerns continue for several weeks, you may wish to contact your doctor or speak with one of the health-care professionals from the treatment team.

Consistent and Persistent

The health-care professionals involved in your child's care will be eager to support your authority in managing the specific behaviors that maintain your child's eating disorder. The treatment team will encourage you to be consistent and persistent, ensuring your child sticks to meals plans, schedules, and activity levels.

However, being consistent may be hard when you are feeling discouraged. This may not be the only thing happening in your life. There may be other children who require your attention, extended family members in need, and issues at work. All of this can make the task of maintaining rules and expectations difficult.

Consensus and Coordination

If you are parenting together with your spouse, partner, or another adult family member, you will need to coordinate your plan so you are not working against each other. One common dynamic in parenting teams is for one parent to respond to the other parent's strictness by becoming more

CASE STUDY Jessica

My mother taught me that you could not take care of anyone if you did not take care of yourself first. It was important to take care of yourself. Things like taking a bath, taking time to read the morning paper, calling a friend…it didn't have to take up much time or space. Little things added up.

Seeing my mom do it, made it easier! She was my role model when it came to working on my self-esteem with my therapist. I was beginning to understand how important it was to take care of me.

continued on page 258

lenient; conversely, the strict parent responds to the leniency by becoming stricter. Neither parent's response alone is likely to be as effective in changing a pattern of eating disordered symptoms as a united parental response.

Working on Your Own

If you are parenting on your own, you may need to seek out a sounding board (friend, adult family member, or counselor) so you do not feel alone in your parenting tasks. As your skills and resources develop, you will feel more confident and in charge.

Support and Comfort

Along with rules and expectations, parents need to provide support and comfort. When everything you offer is rejected, it may be hard to stick with the task of listening to your son or daughter and understanding how they feel. Conversely, your son or daughter will need courage to share with you what they are feeling and what they may need from you.

Often, both of you will be confused by the 'logic' of the eating disorder. For example, you may be perplexed when your child argues with you about eating the smallest amount of food, perhaps one strawberry. Your child is equally confused, recognizing, on the one hand, that the whole discussion about eating is odd, but feeling, on the other hand, that eating the strawberry is somehow wrong. Another time, your child may admit, "I feel isolated and confused. I know my family is suffering, but I can't help it…I feel safer when I follow the rules of my eating disorder. I don't trust myself to just let this go." Your child will need to be comforted when feeling torn like this.

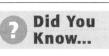 **Did You Know…**

- Good resources for parents, if available in your community, are parent skills groups, parent support groups, or family psychoeducation specifically for parents of children with eating disorders.

- Parents have identified the most powerful support system is speaking with other parents who are presently experiencing a similar situation or have gone through the same process.

Being perplexed by the eating disorder is something you and your child will share. Listening so that you understand your child's eating disorder 'logic' is not easy and will take time, practice, and perhaps professional help.

Balancing Act

Striking a balance between your expectations and limits, on the one hand, and your support and comfort, on the other, will create a strong base for your child to develop the motivation to change the eating disorder behaviors. This will at times be a tough balancing act.

When emphasizing expectations and limits or consequences, your child may accuse you of not being supportive. For example, you might find yourself saying, "If you can't complete this meal, you won't have had enough to eat today. If you don't have enough to eat, then you can't have as much activity. So, we won't be walking the dog together tonight." Your child's response might be, "Walking the dog with you is the only time when I'm happy, when I don't think about food and weight." No doubt, there will be a part of you that wants to waver in favor of giving the kind of support that your child is requesting. Nevertheless, try to hold onto the concept of expectation and consequence, as this will be important during these challenging times.

HOW SHOULD OUR FAMILY TALK ABOUT THE PROBLEM?

A common problem for families of children or adolescents with an eating disorder is how to talk with them and how to talk about the eating disorder with concerned relatives and friends. Here are some frequently asked questions and suggestions addressing this concern.

Q: My daughter has an eating disorder and she seems to be getting better. She looks a lot healthier. But when I tell her how wonderful she looks, she gets angry with me and stomps off. She won't talk about it. I'm not sure what I've done to hurt her feelings. What's going on?

A: When your daughter hears that she is starting to look "better" or "healthier" or "great," it can stir up feelings about her body. Some adolescents with eating disorders may interpret this as meaning, "I don't look as thin as I used to, and if I'm not that thin, then I'm too fat and I should start controlling what I eat again." Another adolescent may understand it to mean, "If I look great now, does that mean I didn't look good before?" It is normal for you to want to show that you care about your daughter. Try to stay focused on her improvement in overall wellness, rather than on her physical appearance. You might try saying, "It's great to be able to spend time together" or "It's nice to see you smiling again."

Q: What should I say to other family members and friends?

A: When you are ready, telling a relative or friend about your child's eating disorder may be appropriate and helpful, but be sure to discuss this with your child. Keeping the problem secret can be disruptive to extended family relationships and friendships — and problematic for siblings.

A common experience for parents is to hear from their own siblings or their own parents comments such as, "Why won't she just eat?" This can sometimes be followed by, "Send her over to my house. I'm sure she'll eat with me."

Take this opportunity to educate your extended family. Eating disorders are complex disorders that are often misunderstood. Some parents find sharing articles about the experience of having a child with an eating disorder or sitting down and watching a video about eating disorders with their children, their own siblings, and their own parents can be a good starting point for conversations and for answering questions. Just as open, direct, and honest communication is helpful in talking with your teen, so it is in talking with your family members.

Different people have different comfort levels about sharing personal information. Often a teen will state a preference that no one should be told anything. Over time, this request may become unrealistic. Discussing the dilemma with your teen and other immediate family members may be helpful. Seek consensus about who should know and what information should be shared.

Generally, friends and relatives are making inquiries because they are worried. Often a simple, confident statement will help them know that their grandchild, niece or nephew, cousin, or friend is getting the help they need.

Keeping your child's illness a secret may stop you from getting the support that comes from speaking to trusted friends, family members, or colleagues. Finding a way to acknowledge your child's concerns about "everyone knowing" and accessing the support you need is important.

You may need to take charge of this situation by telling your child about who needs to be informed, why they need to be informed, and what information they need to have. Discussions about maintaining privacy for you, your family, and your child are of the utmost importance. There is seldom a need "for everyone to know everything."

Q: Friends of my other children and teachers at school are asking if anything is wrong with their sister. What can I advise them to say?

A: Initially, your child may request total privacy, asking that your family tells no one about the eating disorder. This request can become unrealistic for many reasons. Your child may have frequent absences from school to attend health-care appointments or require an admission to hospital. Although your daughter may not be able to acknowledge this, she may be showing physical signs of weight loss that will be noticeable to those around her.

Siblings will need direction from you as to what to say. If a sibling is asked by teachers about their sister's absences, for example, a simple statement like this should suffice: "My sister has an eating disorder and she is away from school now so she can get treatment."

CASE STUDY Brad

Every year for the past 10 years, Brad's mother would go on what she called "the girls' weekend." She had never missed this chance to unwind and commiserate with her three closest friends. They would talk about their husbands, children, parents, and friends. It was a great gab session. She loved it. However, this year it seemed to be impossible for her to go, given what was happening with Brad. She knew her friends would understand.

A week before the scheduled trip, she couldn't help feeling down in the dumps. When her husband asked her what was wrong, she told him. "I can't go on my weekend with the girls. Brad won't eat with anyone but me. What if he stopped eating while I was away? I couldn't forgive myself. It really is too much responsibility to put on someone else."

He felt like he could manage the weekend with Brad and insisted that she go on her trip. He would work with her to develop a plan regarding Brad's eating. It might not be perfect, but the goal was to keep Brad safe. Brad's stepfather felt strongly that his wife should take care of herself and not burn out. What good would she be to Brad if she was exhausted! She needed time to replenish herself, and a weekend away was just what the doctor ordered. This made sense.

Brad's mom went off with her friends for the weekend…anxiously. She surprised herself by having a great time. She checked in regularly at home and was reassured that things were fine. Brad and his stepfather decided that they would have a "boys' weekend" while his mom was away. Brad's mom came back refreshed and ready to fight the battle. Her husband was right.

continued on page 279

CHAPTER 18

Looking for Help from Friends

Anyone who has parented or worked with teenagers knows how important friendships are to an adolescent. During this time, friends become a much larger part of your child's life and have a larger effect on how they feel about themselves. Friends begin to replace you as the most important people in your child's life. These are the 'other' people your children choose to be in their lives.

Adolescents choose their friends for a variety of reasons. Sometimes they are chosen because of common interests, like sports, movies, academic interest, or hobbies. Then again, friends may be chosen for emotional reasons, such as their ability to be supportive. Friends are people whom your child interacts with in school, at camp, or on the soccer field.

Friends help adolescents explore their individuality. Adolescents learn from their friends and their friends learn from them. They can influence what your children wear, how they speak, and what they eat. Friends can influence your children in positive and negative ways.

Friendly Problems

Friends can pose problems for children with eating orders that you can help to solve.

Fitting In

The wish to belong or the desire to 'fit in' with a specific group of friends can sometimes be a trigger for an adolescent to become focused on physical appearance — body shape, weight, and size. Research in this area has shown that young people who spend time together in the same peer group have similar feelings and thoughts about body image, levels of dieting, and other extreme weight loss behaviors.

For instance, if your child is hanging out with friends who

? Did You Know...

• Friends are very important in the life of an adolescent with an eating disorder.

• The dynamics of friendship can trigger an eating disorder; they can also help in the process of recovery.

only value 'skinny' girls, your child may worry about how her friends view her body size. If all your child's friends are dieting, it might be hard for your daughter to resist this behavior. These types of situations can be strong motivators for your child to engage in abnormal eating attitudes and behaviors.

Some teens struggle to fit in. They become overwhelmed at the thought of socializing with teens their own age, although may feel more comfortable in social situations with people who are older or younger. Some adolescents are uncomfortable in any social situation. The total preoccupation with food, weight, and body size may act to protect adolescents with an eating disorder from having to think about their social struggles. Difficulties with making or maintaining friends can be an issue for your child with an eating disorder, especially if this has been a long-standing problem.

Sometimes adolescents need help with learning how to handle individual friends and manage in a group of friends as part of their recovery from their eating disorder. A therapeutic group process might be recommended by your treatment team as one way of helping your son or daughter to begin developing the necessary skills to cope in a social situation.

Bullying and Teasing

Because teasing and bullying behavior is increasingly more common, health-care professionals who work with adolescents with eating disorders will ask about possible incidents of this disturbing behavior by family members or peers.

Dating

Dating raises many new issues for adolescents and their parents. Adolescents face the challenge of developing new social and interpersonal skills with their partner. They also face making decisions about their sexual attitudes and behaviors. Dating can provide companionship.

For some adolescents with eating disorders, these challenges can be overwhelming. They may choose to protect themselves from undergoing these normal developmental changes by shielding themselves from dating, presenting themselves as less attractive to a group of friends or a prospective partner. They may try to lose more weight to become 'invisible' to avoid a romantic relationship. These young people may become even more focused on their weight and eating disordered behaviors to avoid thinking about the pressures associated with dating.

> **? Did You Know...**
>
> • Teasing or bullying (and not only about weight-related issues) may trigger an eating disorder in a vulnerable adolescent.
>
> • Dating can increase awareness about appearance and trigger a desire to be more attractive.

CASE STUDY Jessica

I was on MSN on the computer almost every night. I met Clara on MSN. She was easy to talk to. We had something in common…she was trying to lose weight, too! We compared notes about the latest and greatest tricks to lose weight. We exchanged ideas about what worked and what didn't. I always learned a lot from her. We were friends.

I told Clara about the great talk I had with my dad. I told her that I felt supported and connected. She was happy for me but persisted on talking about weight loss. I couldn't help but get wrapped up in this weight loss conversation once again. I was soon planning my next dieting technique. This one was going to work.

As usual, my mother was hovering around my computer as I was "MSNing" Clara. She must have been reading over my shoulder because she told my dad what I was planning.

My dad and I had another talk. This one was short. We talked about how it wasn't helpful for me to be talking to Clara on MSN. We talked about the best way to approach this issue with Clara. He encouraged me to tell her that I wasn't interested in dieting and that maybe we could talk about other things.

Clara wasn't interested, and over time we stopped talking. I miss her but it's better for me not to be talking about dieting all the time.

continued on page 280

Friendly Solutions

Friends can also play a very important role in supporting the adolescent who has or is recovering from an eating disorder. Tolerance and understanding from your child's friends are especially important. Your child's friends should be supportive and caring. They should be encouraged to listen, not give advice unless asked, and not be disappointed if their advice (when asked for) is ignored.

Encourage your child to maintain their valued friendships. Friends can be most helpful in the process of recovery.

Honest Communication

Friends should be encouraged to be open and honest about their concerns for an adolescent who is struggling with an eating disorder. Friends need to be reminded that they should not make promises they can't keep. For example, "I promise I won't tell anyone you have bulimia nervosa" or "I promise I won't tell your mother that you haven't eaten in 5 days." In fact, friends need to know that it's okay to tell a trusted adult

— parent, teacher, coach, or school nurse — about their concerns for a friend who may have an eating disorder. This way the adolescent with an eating disorder can get professional help as soon as possible. Friends need to know this is not an act of betraying their friend.

No Judgments

Most teens with eating disorders express worry that their peers will judge them, especially about their weight and body image. They are very sensitive about comments regarding their appearance and are renowned for misinterpreting them. For example, an apparently complimentary remark, such as "You look great," can sometimes be interpreted to mean, "You look like you've gained weight" or "You look fat."

Friends should avoid making comments about the adolescent's appearance. The most helpful way to support adolescents struggling with an eating disorder is to express genuine concern about their well-being or provide compliments about their successes and accomplishments. For example, "It's nice to see you having fun with us" or "Congratulations on making the basketball team."

Rejoining Peer Groups

This is a wonderful opportunity for your child's friends to model sensible eating attitudes and behaviors, moderate exercise, and positive self-esteem. Peer group activities that focus on food, body weight, shape or size, and exercise can be stressful. Keep the interactions safe and comfortable.

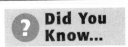

Did You Know...

• Reintegration into their peer group can be a milestone in the recovery of a child or adolescent with an eating disorder.

• Recovery can be strongly influenced by the desire to resume previously enjoyed friendships and related activities.

CASE STUDY Martha

When Martha was recovering from her eating disorder, she met Ted. He soon became her boyfriend. She spent all her time with him, but her parents were not so sure they liked him. She was staying out late, missing curfew, coming home drunk, and her school marks were dropping. It was hard to know what to do. Was this the eating disorder or was it teenage behavior? Was there something else going on?

They didn't think her relationship with Ted was healthy. They wanted to suggest that she end this relationship with Ted but were frightened that this would make her feel worse and perhaps get sicker.

continued on page 269

FREQUENTLY ASKED QUESTIONS

Parents and friends of children and adolescents with eating disorders have many questions about the role of friends in the recovery process. Some of the more common questions are posed and answered here.

Q: **Our daughter has a number of close friends who used to hang out with her before the eating disorder was diagnosed. What do we tell her friends now?**

A: Sharing information about your child's eating disorder with friends can be a complicated matter. Some young people are quite comfortable letting their friends know that they have an eating disorder. Others are adamant that nobody, including their friends, know.

Disguising the eating disorder is not easy. Adolescents usually know when their friends are sick with an eating disorder, especially when their friend is hospitalized after having lost a significant amount of weight.

If your child still wants to keep the eating disorder a secret, discuss the implications of sharing versus not sharing this information with friends. You might want to highlight specific issues that could present problems if the disorder is kept a secret. For instance, most adolescents participate in social events that include food, such as eating at a friend's house, going to a movie or party, and meeting for dinner at a restaurant. Avoiding these occasions will not go unnoticed by friends. Depending on the meal plan, your child also may need to eat a larger quantity of food than her healthy friends. Having to eat large quantities of food at school or other social events likewise will not go unnoticed by friends.

If the eating disorder is kept a secret, your son or daughter may place themselves in the awkward position of having to dodge questions or to explain these odd behaviors. Concealing this information from friends can present a new set of problems.

Remind your child that friends can be sympathetic and supportive, not always judgmental. Help your child to understand that being honest, open, and sincere with friends is advisable. Also let your child's friends know that their friend will most likely recover from this illness, more quickly with the support of friends like them.

Q: My 14-year-old daughter's best friend came to talk to me because she is concerned that our daughter has an eating disorder. This friend tried to talk to our daughter and express her concerns…but she got very angry. What should we do?

A: This can be a very difficult situation. First, it is admirable to know that your daughter's best friend is concerned about her. It is also commendable that her best friend tried to talk with your daughter about her concerns. Being supportive and caring, but not confrontational, is important.

Friends shouldn't try to take this on by themselves. Your daughter's best friend is truly a wonderful friend to be able to share her concerns with an adult who is in a position to intervene.

Q: Should we let friends visit our child while she is in the hospital? Can this create problems?

A: Many parents wonder whether this is a good idea. On the one hand, friends can offer support; on the other, they may make your child feel even more uncomfortable. You and your child will need to agree that visiting friends will have a positive influence. Be sure to speak to your treatment team about this issue. Their experience in dealing with this question should be helpful.

Q: While undergoing treatment, our daughter has made friends with other kids suffering from eating disorders. We fear she may be learning 'tricks of the trade' from them. Should we discourage these friendships?

A: There is no one 'right' answer to this question. Teens with eating disorders may be able to support one another to be healthy in a way that families and professionals or even other friends cannot. It can be extremely helpful for some adolescents who are struggling with their eating disorder to know that there are others with similar feelings and conflicts. There may be comfort for your child in knowing that she is not alone. Positive, supportive friendships at a stage when the adolescent is ready to think about recovery can be very helpful.

On the other hand, you should also be aware that others might negatively influence your child if they are supporting her to remain sick. First, talk with your child about this relationship. In addition, discuss this relationship with your treatment team. If it is clear that the friendship in question is harmful to your child, your response should be consistent with your response to other eating disordered behaviors and attitudes. That is, limit the contact when possible and encourage the development of positive, supportive friendships with others.

Q: We suspect that our son has developed an unhealthy friendship with an Internet 'friend' that may impede his recovery. What should we do?

A: Some adolescents, especially those who have become isolated from their friends, may turn to 'cyberfriends' found on the Internet. Others may become involved in Internet chat rooms for eating disordered people. Young people with eating disorders may also discover "pro-ana" (anorexia) or "pro-mia" (bulimia) websites. These sites contain harmful information geared toward maintaining the illness that may negatively influence your child's struggle with an eating disorder. Treat this 'friend' the way you do the illness. Ask your treatment team for help.

Q: We're not sure how to discuss our child's condition with our friends and close acquaintances. What should we tell them?

A: As you try to cope with the impact of your child's eating disorder on your own life, it is very important for you to seek support and solace, not only from your family members and your health-care professionals, but also from your own friends.

Admitting to a friend that your child has an eating disorder is not an easy task. You may fear that your friends will judge you as a poor parent, perhaps not worthy of their friendship. In most cases, this fear is misplaced. Good friends can be an important source of support. They can offer a sympathetic listening ear. They can help out with car pools, babysitting, and making meals, giving you some time for yourself. Let your friends know how they can help. Do you need a break after working all day? Do you need someone to listen to you without giving opinions? Do you need an opinion? Be clear with your friends about what you would find helpful, so that they know how to best support you.

With their good humor and view of the brighter side of things, friends can distract you from the daily challenges of dealing with a child with an eating disorder.

How parents behave with their friends provides a role model for children and adolescents in dealing with their friends. Be honest and direct with your friends. Let your child know that you are asking your friends for help. Explain about how important it is for you to get help and support from your own friends. Your child may decide to do the same.

Help for Judging Friendships

Whether your child benefits or suffers from a particular friendship with another young person with an eating disorder depends on several important issues:

1. Does your child's friend support your child returning to health or does the friend endorse maintaining the illness? The new friend's desire to get better is important in encouraging your child to get better as well.
2. Is your son or daughter ready to cope with someone else's illness as well as their own? Your child may gain strength from helping a new friend with an eating disorder to make a change, but beware that this friendship may be draining if your child has to carry two loads, with the friend becoming dependent.
3. Where is your child with respect to the process of change? If your child is precontemplative — that is, not even ready to consider getting better — friendships with other eating disordered children or adolescents might be less helpful than at a contemplative or action stage, when your child is either thinking about recovery or actually taking steps toward better health.

Help your daughter or son to identify the friends that they feel comfortable knowing about the eating disorder. For some teens, this may be a couple of close friends, while for others it might include all their friends. You might also discuss what it might be like if your daughter or son is included in social events related to food and how they might manage this if friends are not aware of the issues involved.

HELP FOR HANDLING FRIENDS

This friendly advice from health-care professionals and fellow parents of children with eating disorders may help you in solving any problems concerning the role of friends in your child's recovery.

Do

- **Do** talk with your child about whether or not they want to share information about the eating disorder with other people.

- **Do** support positive friendships that facilitate your child's recovery. Encourage your child to maintain these healthy, supportive friendships. Friendships should be safe and comfortable.

- **Do** be gentle and caring in expressing your concerns about the eating attitudes and behaviors of your child's friends. You do not want to appear to be judging their behavior or condemning them.

- **Do** encourage your child to participate in peer group activities that do not focus on food, body weight, shape, or size. But if the occasion arises, help your child to plan strategies for managing food issues in social situations.

- **Do** help your child to reintegrate into their peer group so as to resume old friendships and previously enjoyed social activities. Your child may begin to model the sensible eating attitudes, moderate exercise, and positive self-esteem shown by friends.

- **Do** let your child's friends know how they can help, with your child's permission, of course. They will want to help but may not know how. Be clear about what your child needs from friends.

- **Do** let your own friends know how they can help. Your friends will want to help but don't necessarily know how. Be clear about what you need.

- **Do** reach out for the support you need. Talk to family members, friends, support groups, or get professional help. Your friends and family members can be an important source of support.

Don't

- **Don't** permit 'negative' friendships that encourage your child to maintain the eating disorder. Don't be critical of your child's friends, but establish limits and restrictions to protect your child's health.

- **Don't** let your child avoid social situations because of concerns around food-related issues. Avoiding these situations may drive your child into further isolation from family and friends.

- **Don't** confront your child about eating behaviors in front of friends. Embarrassing your child will only compound the problem.

- **Don't** resist help and support from friends and family. Don't let pride of fear get in the way.

- **Don't** underestimate the importance of your child's friendships.

CASE STUDY Susan

Susan had done well when she returned to the Day Treatment Program. She was soon well enough to be discharged. She was going back to school after having been away for almost 7 months.

But she was worried about what everyone would say. Would anyone still be her friend? Although she had stayed in contact with some of her friends and knew how excited they were about her coming back to school, she was terrified. She looked so different…what would people say? She had missed so much…how was she ever going to catch up?

Her father reminded her that people would likely lose interest in her story after a few minutes. Most people were "the stars in their own show."

Prior to her discharge from the Day Treatment Program, Susan, her parents, and her therapist talked a lot about the different types of questions that her friends and teachers might have. They 'role played' and prepared Susan for these questions. This was great preparation for what was to come!

Susan anxiously returned to school. Her parents and therapist were right. It was much easier than she thought. People asked her where she had been and she answered them honestly. She told them that she had an eating problem and lost a lot of weight. She was doing much better now and was ready to get on with things. Most people responded by telling her that they were glad to see her back. Quickly, the conversations moved to important topics like friends, movies, and parties.

continued on page 276

CHAPTER 19

Preventing Eating Disorders by Educating Teachers, Coaches, and Counselors

A recent trend in the primary prevention (before any negative behaviors are present) of disordered eating involves adopting health promotion programs designed to develop overall wellness, as well as alter some of the predisposing risk factors related to disordered eating, such as low self-esteem and perfectionism.

Helping young people build positive self-esteem and enjoy healthy, active lifestyles, without developing a fear of food, has replaced the more traditional approach of highlighting negative, problem-based issues that may unintentionally glamorize eating disorders, provide techniques for controlling weight control, and introduce negative language about some kinds of food.

These prevention programs are not only effective in the home, but also at school, in sports, and at summer camps. You can help to promote these prevention programs by bringing them to the attention of teachers, coaches, and counselors, if they have not already been trained in preventing eating disorders.

Confusing Messages

Public health concerns about the increasing prevalence of childhood obesity and associated chronic medical conditions have coincided with prevention strategies designed to promote healthy eating and active living. On the one hand, these health promotion strategies can help set the stage for the development of healthy lifestyles. On the other, emphasizing weight issues has the potential to trigger the onset of eating disorders among some children, fueling existing preoccupations with body image and weight among those at risk. Your child may be hearing mixed messages.

While childhood obesity can be a legitimate concern, limiting or restricting the amount of food available to children can backfire. For example, disrupting a child's internal cues for hunger and satiety (feeling full) can initiate a cycle of dieting, weight gain, and low self-esteem. They may resort to cutting back on certain foods, skipping meals, restricting calories, or using food supplements and other medications (including steroids) for the purposes of weight loss or muscle gain.

This mixed message is compounded by what they see and hear in the media. On the one hand, they are bombarded with unrealistic (and often unattainable) images of excessively thin and exaggerated muscular body shapes, which they are led to believe can be attained through fad diets and exercise regimes. On the other hand, they are targeted by advertisements enticing them to eat high-fat, fast foods and other unhealthy food products.

Sorting out these confusing messages is the fundamental step in preventing eating disorders. Although some children might require professional advice to help them achieve or maintain a healthy weight, exposing children to healthy eating, active living, and size acceptance through practice and role modeling is the best approach.

PREVENTION PROGRAMS

Programs for preventing eating disorders now focus on three strategies. Research has shown that this approach helps to boost body satisfaction and global self-esteem, while reducing unhealthy dieting.

1. Promoting healthy eating and active living, focusing on non-dieting approaches to eating and physical activity.

2. Developing media literacy to think critically how (for example, using computers to enhance photographs of models) and why (to increase product sales) the media convey their messages, especially as they apply to images of beauty, fitness, shape, size, success, and happiness.

3. Learning life skills, including ways to develop positive body image and self-esteem; to cope with stress through such strategies as assertive communication; to combat weight-based teasing and peer pressures to diet; and to develop positive interpersonal relationships.

Q: In my daughter's physical education class, the teacher posted the students' weights on the wall and organized a contest to see who could lose the most amount of weight in one week. Is this healthy?

A: This is what you might consider thinking about or doing. Because of recent concerns about childhood obesity, increased attention is being given to measuring children's weight. In their attempts to improve students' health, teachers might inadvertently select activities that promote weight and shape preoccupation among children (measuring and posting weights), who otherwise might not be thinking about it.

This approach is especially dangerous for children and adolescents recovering from an eating disorder, given that treatment programs discourage measuring body weight or shape as a way to decrease weight or shape preoccupation.

School-wide approaches that foster healthy lifestyles among all children, regardless of their body size or shape, prevent the stigmatizing of larger children and encourage all students, including thin children, to engage in healthy eating and active living practices.

? Did You Know...

• School-based education programs are now recommended to refrain from teaching children and adolescents about eating disorders.

• Teaching the topic of eating disorders is ineffective for improving eating attitudes and behaviors and may actually encourage some young people to experiment with newly-learned behaviors, such as laxative use, self-induced vomiting, and excessive exercise.

School

Schools are an ideal setting to offer effective prevention techniques because of the access to a wide variety of young people.

These programs have been initiated with children in late elementary school in response to the normative onset of body image concerns and disordered eating during young adolescence. These concerns are often spurred on by the physical changes associated with puberty, an increase in the desire for peer acceptance, and the onset of romantic interests — all of which heighten their awareness of physical appearance and attractiveness.

The goal of the prevention strategies is to boost resilience by helping youth adjust or bounce back from the changes brought on by stressful events associated with the early adolescence transition. The goal is to minimize the likelihood of these young people adopting restrictive dieting or other unhealthy body change strategies as ways to cope with this stressful life transition.

EVERY BODY IS A SOMEBODY

"Every BODY is a Somebody" is an active learning educational program for promoting healthy body image, positive self-esteem, healthy eating, and an active lifestyle for adolescent females. This program focuses on the promotion of media literacy and life skills — for example, ways to promote positive body image and self-esteem; ways to adopt a non-dieting approach to healthy eating and active living; information about the genetic influences on overall body shape; stress management skills, such as assertive communication; and skills to build positive relationships and to cope with peer pressures to diet. The facilitators' guide provides background information and practical activities that can be carried out in the classroom or peer group settings. This guide is available at: www.bodyimagecoalition.org

CASE STUDY Martha

Martha's physical education class was doing an assignment on healthy living. Martha felt like she was an expert on this subject… after all she had attended psychoeducation sessions at the Eating Disorder Program.

However, she was terrified when she learned that during the next class everyone would have their height and weight measured. To top it off, everyone in the class would have to determine their body mass index (BMI) and decide whether they were "just right," "at risk for being overweight," or "overweight"…and then report back to the class.

Martha was so horrified that she decided to drop physical education. There was just no way she was going to be weighed in public, in front of all her classmates. She went to the guidance department, filled out the form to drop the course, and forged her parent's signature. She decided not to tell anyone. If her parents knew, they would make a big fuss! Her parents might even ask her to educate everyone about why this was not okay. She couldn't imagine doing any of this. She hated the thought of having all this attention focus on her…an eating disorder poster child. She just wanted to be a normal kid.

continued on page 279

Teacher Training

These prevention initiatives require teachers to have curriculum support and access to up-to-date resources that are matched to the education expectations. When teachers deliver body image, healthy eating, and lifestyle information to students, 'how' is just as important as 'what.' Particular attention needs to be given to the teacher's method of delivery.

For this reason, it is crucial that teachers receive in-service training to learn how their own personal values and beliefs about food, weight, and shape can have an influence on those of their students. In particular, if teachers model or talk about fad diets or make negative comments about the way other people look, students might follow suit.

In the same way, some of the methods used to teach nutrition (e.g., calorie counting and analyzing food labels) might inadvertently increase weight and shape preoccupation among some children, particularly those at risk of, or recovering from, an eating disorder.

In addition to teachers receiving in-service training on primary prevention strategies that can be implemented in the classroom setting, school support staff (social workers, youth counselors, and psychologists) can learn how to assess, intervene early, or refer at-risk students, where appropriate, to local specialized eating disorder services.

Training on the assessment, prevention, and treatment of eating disorders is offered by such agencies as the Ontario Community Outreach Program for Eating Disorders (416-430-4051 or 800-463-1856 within Ontario, Canada).

HEALTH-AT-ANY-SIZE

Educating teachers, through involvement in school councils or direct parent-teacher communication, about the dangers of weight management techniques might be useful. You may also want to inform your child's school that the World Health Organization (WHO) encourages the health-at-any-size approach, which is a health-centered, rather than weight-centered, approach, focusing on the whole person — physically, mentally, and socially. This approach shifts the focus to active living, healthy eating, respecting each individual, and promoting health and well-being for all, regardless of size. Health-at-any-size supports appropriate lifestyle behavior changes to achieve these objectives.

Peer Support Groups

Within the school, peer groups can have a significant influence on a child's or adolescent's body image or eating behavior. In fact, through talk, modeling of behavior, and teasing, the peer environment can create a subculture that has the ability to exaggerate weight-loss strategies. Girls who feel pressured to diet or who are teased about their weight and shape may experience negative body image or disordered eating.

Peers groups can also be valuable in preventing and treating eating disorders. Peer support groups have been piloted in the school setting and have been shown to improve the eating attitudes and behaviors of young teen girls. It is thought that the participants of these peer groups benefit from having the opportunity to problem-solve issues related to peer pressures within the safety of a small intimate group.

School-Wide Policies

Other important school-wide strategies that can be implemented include policies against weight-based teasing and sexual harassment, guidelines against the use of 'starve-a-thons' as fundraising techniques, allocation of adequate space and time for lunch and snacks, awareness of lunchroom talk that promotes unhealthy eating, and the replacement of fat-caliper testing and group weigh-ins with the promotion of physical activity that includes students of all sizes, shapes, and skill levels.

As a family, you may also choose to adopt family-wide healthy eating and active living policies.

HELP FOR PROMOTING POSITIVE BODY IMAGE

Share with your child's teacher, coach, or camp counselor the following tips on ways to promote positive body image and healthy eating.

- Help students to know that, as part of normal growth, especially during puberty, their weight and body fat percentage will increase. There is no need to worry about these natural changes or to be ashamed of them.

- Discourage restrictive forms of dieting because, paradoxically, restriction is linked to weight gain. The eating behaviors students may practice in the attempt to lose weight lead to the opposite result. Advise students that any form of dieting, unless directed by their doctor, is unhealthy, perhaps dangerous.

- Create realistic images about overall body shape given the evidence that genetic factors account for part of the variance in body mass index (BMI). Not everyone can or should look the same. Encourage and model respect for diversity in weight and shape.

- Teach students to think critically about the unrealistic and unhealthy messages concerning physical appearance, dieting, and eating behavior that appear in the media, especially images of ideal body shapes and claims for the effectiveness of fad diets.

- Model not only the physical but also the emotional benefits of physical activity. Be careful not to encourage over-activity, though.

- Recognize the negative impact of weight-based teasing by peers on the body satisfaction and emotional health of children. Teasing often compounds the problem. Don't let this kind of teasing occur at school, in sports, or at camp.

COMPREHENSIVE AND QUALITY SCHOOL HEALTH PROGRAMS

Comprehensive School Health and Quality School Health are two programs that advocate for school-wide approaches to health promotion focused on improving the health curriculum, the available support services, the social environment, and the physical environment at the school. A number of health-related issues fall under this umbrella, including nutrition and body image; physical education and activity; bullying and violence; mental, emotional, and social health; drug and alcohol use; injury prevention; dental health and sexual health; and chronic disease prevention.

The model's application to the prevention of disordered eating could include, among other things, the following:

Health Curriculum

Classroom education on nutrition. In-service training of teachers on ways to promote size acceptance and prevent body size discrimination in their teaching practices.

Support Services

Access to dietitians or nutritionists in the community in case any students require assessment or nutrition counseling.

Social Environment

Universal, non-stigmatizing school breakfast, snack, and lunch programs. School policies respecting diversity in size and shape.

Physical Environment

Nutritious foods, comfortable space, and adequate time for snacks and meals. Safe food handling.

More information about the Quality School Health program is available at: www.cahperd.ca.

WARNING SIGNS

Teachers can help assist in the prevention or early detection of an eating disorder. Given the secrecy surrounding eating disorders, it is not uncommon for friends to be the first to recognize that something is wrong. Students may also confide in a teacher or guidance counselor about their concern for a friend (or about themselves).

There are several warning signs that teachers may recognize among students that indicate an eating problem. Be alert if students:

- Overestimate or underestimate their body size.
- Talk about feeling "fat" or "ugly."
- Talk negatively about parts of body.
- Worry about being too small or too large.
- Feel ashamed or embarrassed by their appearance, size, height, or physical maturity.
- "Over do it" with physical activity.
- Practice unusual eating habits.
- Restrict food intake.
- Experience irregular menstrual periods or loss of menstrual periods.
- Show mood swings or irritability.
- Feel guilt or shame about eating.
- Avoid certain foods, particularly those considered "fattening."
- Say they are "fat" when they are not overweight.
- Show noticeable weight loss or frequent weight fluctuation.

Medical Intervention

If school personnel are concerned that a student has lost a considerable amount of weight or appears emotionally or medically unstable, they should encourage the student and family members to seek help from their family doctor or pediatrician. Medical monitoring is important given the secretive nature of eating disorders and the severe symptoms that can, as a result, go unnoticed, such as binge eating or self-induced vomiting.

School personnel can refer to the website for The National Eating Disorder Information Centre to obtain information on how to approach someone who they suspect has an eating disorder (www.nedic.ca).

Resources

Teachers and school support staff might benefit from reading material on eating disorders so as to become familiar with the early warning signs and ways to help a young person seek help for their disorder. For example, The National Eating Disorder Information Centre's *An Introduction to Food and Weight Problems* is especially useful, as is *Understanding and Overcoming an Eating Disorder*. Please see the "Eating Disorder Information Resources" section of this book for more information on this topic.

If communication is facilitated between the school personnel and the health-care professionals working within the eating disorder program, the health-care team can coach teachers and school support staff on ways to ease the student's transition back to school once they are discharged from a treatment program.

Special considerations may be necessary for these when considering their re-involvement in physical activity or sport at school, or their participation in activities related to nutrition. Teaching methods used to help prevent childhood obesity might inadvertently interfere with the progress of a child's recovery from an eating disorder.

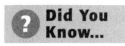

Did You Know...

- If resources are available, trained school support staff can facilitate early intervention programs for students at risk, reaching them before their eating disorder symptoms worsen and motivating them to seek professional treatment outside of the school setting, if need be.

Sports

Choosing a sport or physical activity for your child requires some careful planning. Unfortunately, many sport environments today have stringent standards regarding body size and overall physical appearance. Some coaches might suggest, either directly or indirectly, that a particular body shape or size is required for children to participate or to continue to participate in the activity or sport. If that recommended body shape conflicts with the child's natural size, this might encourage the adoption of unhealthy body change strategies.

This focus compromises the enjoyment of the activity and, in some instances, can trigger body image concerns among children.

Q: My 12-year-old daughter's skating coach brought a scale to skating practice sessions and said that he plans to weigh the girls from now on, since they are going through puberty and he does not want them to gain weight. What should I do?

A: Consider planning a meeting with your daughter's coach or sharing an article explaining how girls experience natural increases in weight and body fat during puberty. Help the coach understand that some increase in weight might also be attributed to a gain in muscle generated from working out, particularly among children involved in elite sports.

Growth experienced by children and teens necessitates increased amounts of energy and nutrients from a wide variety of foods to help with optimal muscle and bone growth (especially if they are very active). If normal growth is interrupted by malnutrition (imposed weigh-ins may trigger dieting out of fear of weight gain), particularly in combination with excessive exercise, the athlete's performance and overall health will be compromised.

Talk with other parents to see if you can form a committee within the sport setting to raise awareness about these health issues. Be sure to inquire about the instructor's or coach's overall philosophy before enrolling your child in a sports activity. This can be done by interviewing the coach or speaking to other parents whose children are enrolled in that activity. Next, observe your son or daughter when they first take part in the activity. Are the children all having fun? Does the activity include children of varying body sizes and shapes? Is the focus of the coach's instruction and feedback on skill and ability rather than on the child's appearance?

BODYSENSE

The BODYSENSE pilot program is dedicated to the promotion of positive body image in sports settings for athletes with the ultimate goal of preventing disordered eating. The program deals with people who are already at risk of developing disordered eating — female athletes. Discussion groups are held in club settings, and prevention information is available in brochures, newsletters, and guidelines at: www.bodysense.ca

CASE STUDY Susan

Before Susan got sick, she attended a weekly dance class. Jaime was Susan's friend from dance class. Jaime's mother, Lisa, called Susan's mother one night. Lisa asked if Susan would come to the dance class and talk about her eating disorder. Susan's mother was shocked at the request. It seemed rather insensitive.

She obviously had no idea what Susan was going through. Susan's mother tried to be polite. She wondered why Lisa was asking Susan to do this. Over the course of the discussion, Susan's mother realized that Lisa was worried about Jaime and some of the other girls in the dance class. There was a new dance instructor who was very concerned about body shape and weight. He told the class, "To be a great dancer, you must have the 'right' body type." He continued, "I don't think it would be a good idea for anyone to gain any weight at this time and it may be advantageous to even shed a few pounds." He also believed that "only the weak developed eating disorders."

Susan's mother began to understand Lisa's request. She made the following suggestions. "Listen Lisa, if you are worried about Jaime, talk to her about your concerns and take her to see your family doctor or pediatrician. I would also recommend that you speak to the head of the dance school and share your concerns about the messages that the girls in the class are getting from the new teacher. Often the local community eating disorder coalition has information and resources on the prevention of eating disorders. That might be helpful for both you and the dance school. We have learned through our reading and treatment that speaking to young girls about eating disorder can often make the situation worse. There are better ways of dealing with this situation."

continued on page 278

Camp

Going to camp, especially overnight camp, is usually an enjoyable way for children and adolescents to gain independence. This also marks a time when children might experience a change in their eating or activity patterns. Some children might exercise more than usual without adjusting their caloric intake, leading to weight loss during a period of rapid physical growth. Other children may be influenced by the eating patterns of their fellow campers or of their camp counselors.

Given the age group of most camp counselors, some might be engaging in dieting or experimenting with their own eating, adopting a vegetarian lifestyle, cutting back on certain foods, or worrying about their body image, for example. This could result in young campers making significant changes to their own pattern of eating, changes that may go unnoticed until the child returns home from camp.

Through a discussion with the camp director, you might find out if there are any policies about nutrition, eating, and physical activity. You might also inquire if the counselors who work at your child's camp undergo training about eating disorders, including how their own eating attitudes and behaviors might influence their campers and how to recognize the early warning signs of an eating disorder.

CHAPTER 20

Understanding the Long and Hard Journey to Recovery

Throughout this book we have followed the case histories of several young people with eating disorders — Susan, Martha, Brad, and Jessica. We have also read Tammy's account of the onset of her eating disorder and her courageous recovery. Not everyone has been this fortunate.

What have we learned from these case histories? Let's review the status of each case.

Susan

Susan was almost 18 years old and still not fully recovered from the eating disorder. She was still underweight and her bones showed signs of osteoporosis. The doctors were concerned that her height had been compromised...she was probably shorter than she would have been if this hadn't happened. She was learning to cope with this.

The good news was that she was getting her menstrual period. She was also still in treatment and needed the motivational effects of regular clinic visits. The doctor was clear that if she lost weight, she would need to be readmitted to the hospital. She was also in individual therapy...that 'psychodynamic stuff' was finally making sense and starting to help a lot. Her family still came for some family therapy booster sessions when things got really difficult.

After all these years, it felt like the eating disorder team was part of her family. Her team started talking to her and her family about transition to the adult health-care system. Susan was curious, cautious, and excited, all at the same time. She liked the idea that she would be making all her treatment decisions and that her family would only know things if she gave the adult treatment team her consent. She liked the thought of being treated like a grown-up. Sometimes it felt like everyone in her family treated her like a baby.

But secretly she was terrified. It was safe here in the adolescent eating disorder program. No one would ever let anything bad happen to her. She felt confused. She wasn't quite sure what would happened if all the treatment decisions were left up to her?

She also knew how terrified her parents were about this transition. Her parents worked hard to come to terms with the fact that this chapter in her life -- the pediatric eating disorder treatment — was soon to come to a close and a new chapter was about to begin. They had done everything in their power to help prepare Susan for her adult life. They had some experience with preparation for adulthood with their other children. This, however, was different. It seemed like the eating disorder interfered with this process and made it that much more difficult. Susan would be considered a "young adult" in the adult health-care system. Was she ready? Were they ready? The unknown was frightening.

Brad

It felt like a long time, but Brad slowly recovered. He was in treatment for 18 long months. His parents understood that 18 months of treatment was relatively short in the treatment of an eating disorder. The medication really helped the anxiety disorder and the eating disorder. The therapy was really important, too…talking about feelings, understanding each other, and working together to find solutions.

Working with the dietitian and learning to take baby steps was influential in learning how to eat again. Finally, working on parenting skills was the final nail in the eating disorder's coffin. Things were going to be all right.

Martha

Martha got better slowly. By the time she turned 18, the eating disorder was history. But Martha had a rocky adolescence.

She continued to be a challenge to her parents. Her parents learned to stand firm, set limits, and force her to face the consequences of her behavior.

"With rights came responsibility," her parents would repeat over and over again. This meant that her parents did not bail her out the second time she got caught shoplifting. The eating disorder team also refused to write a letter excusing her because of a mental disorder. She went to court and was required to participate in community service. This incident had a huge impact on her. That was the last time she ever did anything like that again.

Years later, when Martha had her own family, she would reflect on her own adolescence — her anger, changing feelings, fears and hopes. This provided her with some perspective. She recognized the difficulties she caused her parents. Despite all the challenges, they provided her with love, compassion, sensitivity, consistency, positive reinforcement, and understanding. They were always there for her!

Jessica

Over time, with therapy, nutritional counseling, and the support of my family, I stopped binging. The first step was to stop restricting. I focused on real health. I learned to eat normally and to exercise moderately. Mostly, I worked on feeling good about myself.

An unexpected thing happened when I stopped dieting… it was much easier to stop binging, and when I stopped binging, I lost weight. I'm still not thin, not even close, but that's okay. I'm doing everything I can in order to stay healthy.

Some days I feel fat and other days I actually feel beautiful.

Tammy

Tammy's recovery from her eating disorder was a long and hard journey. Despite her chronic illness, multiple treatments, numerous hospitalizations, and relentless feelings of helplessness and despair, Tammy got better. Tammy's story underscores just how devastating and dangerous eating disorders can be. In some cases, they are even life-threatening.

Approximately, 1 in 10 people with child-onset anorexia nervosa die from the eating disorder. Young people die as a result of either suicide or medical complications secondary to starvation. But with the proper treatment and support, teenagers with eating disorders do get better. Like Tammy, it may take some time before a person with an eating disorder learns to live a healthy life.

Tammy's experience highlights some of the most important issues about recovery from an eating disorder. As we have said over and over again, eating disorders are complicated. Recovery from an eating disorder is also a complicated process. Recovery means improvement in a number of aspects of an adolescent's life: weight restoration, eating attitudes and behaviors, menstruation, mental health status, friendships, and family relationships. It is no wonder that recovery is a long, hard process.

4 RECOVERY FACTS ABOUT EATING DISORDERS

Both Tammy's experience with anorexia nervosa and the medical research emphasize a number of important facts.

1. Early recognition of an eating disorder is important. The longer the duration of the illness, the harder it is to achieve recovery. That is why it is so important to diagnose an eating disorder early in the course of the illness.

2. Once an eating disorder is recognized, parents should actively seek treatment. The earlier the intervention, the more likely a child or adolescent with an eating disorder will recover.

3. Like Tammy, most adolescents with eating disorders take a long time to recover. Medical research has shown that early weight restoration for adolescents with anorexia nervosa helps the recovery process. Early discharge from the hospital below a healthy weight often means poorer outcomes and multiple hospitalizations.

4. Full-recovery from anorexia nervosa is achieved by half of teenagers at 6 years of follow-up and by 75% of patients at 10 to 12 years of follow-up. Be patient and don't give up. Young people with this disorder take a long time to get better, but the majority do recover. Other research has shown that the outcome for adolescents with eating disorders has improved over time. For instance, the outcome of an adolescent today is better than it was 30 years ago. This may be due to earlier diagnosis and better treatment.

Remember that each child or adolescent with an eating disorder will experience their own journey to recovery. Some teenagers will recover very quickly, but others will take much longer. Parents need to be prepared for their child's own journey. Parents may face months and sometimes years of treatment, anxiety, and despair. It is not uncommon for parents to feel defeated and helpless during the course of this illness. Patience and perseverance are critical!

Parents of a child or adolescent with an eating disorder may find it difficult and challenging to deal with such a long-term problem. It can be frightening to see your child physically compromised and mentally tormented by these disorders. But remember, most children will recover.

Like Tammy, your child has the ability to win the battle against the eating disorder.

9 STEPS TO RECOVERY

In Tammy's courageous account of her struggle with anorexia nervosa, she generously shares with us her advice. She recognizes that parents play a pivotal role in the recovery of their child and encourages parents to consider these nine important points.

1. Recognize that eating disorders are complex.

2. Learn as much about eating disorders as possible.

3. Understand that young people with eating disorders come in all shapes, weights, and sizes.

4. Keep in mind that the eating disorder is the illness, not the person.

5. Reassure yourself that parents don't cause eating disorders.

6. Work with your children, as well as your children's teachers, coaches, and counselors, to prevent abnormal eating attitudes and behaviors.

7. Support your child in the process of assessing and treating the eating disorder.

8. Don't forget to take care of yourself and your family.

9. Be hopeful even though recovery can be a hard and long process.

Eating Disorder Information Resources

Print Resources

Books

Anorexia Nervosa: A Survival Guide for Families, Friends and Sufferers
by Janet Treasure. London, UK: Psychology Press, 1977.

Beauty Myth
by Naomi Wolfe. New York, NY and Toronto, ON: Random House, 1991.

Body Love
by R. Freedman. New York, NY: Harper & Row, 1988.

Consuming Passions
Edited by Catrina Brown and Karin Jasper. Toronto, ON: Second Story Press, 1993.

Fighting Invisible Tigers: Stress Management Guide for Teens
by E. Hipp. Minneapolis, MN: Free Spirit Publishing, 1995.

Girl Power
by H. Carlip. New York, NY: Warner Books, 1995.

Helping Your Child Overcome an Eating Disorder
by Bethany Teachman, Marlene Schwartz, Bonnie Gordic, and Brenda Coyle. Oakland, CA: New Harbinger Publications, 2003.

Losing It: False Hopes and Fat Profits in the Diet Industry
by L. Fraser. New York, NY: Plume, 1998.

The New Our Bodies Ourselves
by Boston Women's Health Collective. New York, NY: Simon & Shuster, 1984.

The Parent's Guide to Childhood Eating Disorders
by Marcia Herrin and Nancy Matsumoto. New York, NY: Henry Holt, 2002.

Real Gorgeous
by Kaz Cooke. New York, NY: W. W. Norton, 1994.

The Relaxation and Stress Reduction Workbook
by M. Daris, E.R. Eshelman, and M. McKay. Oakland, CA: New Harbinger, 1995.

Reviving Ophelia
by Mary Pipher. New York, NY: Putman, 1994.

Surviving an Eating Disorder: Strategies for Family and Friends
by Michelle Siegel, Judith Brisman, and Margot Weinshel. New York, NY: Harper Perennial, 1997.

When Girls Feel Fat: Helping Girls Through Adolescence
by Sandra Susan Friedman. New York, NY: Harper Collins, 1997.

When Your Child Has an Eating Disorder
by Abigail Natenshon. San Francisco, CA: Jossey-Bass, 1999.

Gurze Books sells books on eating disorders and related topics that are suitable for adolescents and adults. View their website at: www.gurze.com

Magazines

Hues
PO Box 7778, Ann Arbor, MI 48107 e-mail: hues@branson.org

Ms Magazine
PO Box 50008, Boulder, CO 80323-0008

New Moon
PO Box 3587, Duluth, MN 55803-3587

Radiance: The Magazine for Large Women
Created in 1984 and published quarterly for 16 years, this magazine supported women "all sizes of large" living proud, full, active lives, at whatever weight, with self-love and self-respect. Currently not active but back issues are available. Tel: 510-885-1505. Website: www.radiancemagazine.com/index.html

Societies and Associations

Academy for Eating Disorders (AED) is an organization for professionals from all fields who deal with eating disorders. Tel: 847-498-4274. Website: www.aedweb.org.

American Academy of Child and Adolescent Psychiatry (AACAP) is a national professional medical association dedicated to treating and improving the quality of life for children, adolescents, and families affected by mental, behavioral, or developmental disorders. Website: www.aacap.org

American Academy of Pediatrics (AAP) is dedicated to the well-being of all infants, children, adolescents and young adults. Website: www.aap.org

The American Dietetic Association (ADA) has information on good nutrition and sensible eating habits. Tel: 800-877-1600. Website: www.eatright.org

American Psychiatric Association (APA) works to ensure effective treatment for all persons with mental disorders, including mental retardation and substance-related disorders. Tel: 703-907-7300. Website: www.psych.org

Anorexia Nervosa and Related Eating Disorders, Inc. (ANRED) provides information about eating disorders, including self-help tips about recovery and prevention. Website: www.anred.com

The Canadian Paediatric Society (CPS) is committed to the health needs of children and youth. Tel: 613-526-9397. Website: www.caringforkids.cps.ca

Canadian Psychiatric Association (CPA–APC) is dedicated to ensuring the highest possible standard of professional practice in providing psychiatric services to Canadians. Tel: 613-234-2815. Website: www.cpa-apc.org/

Dietitians of Canada has information about good nutrition and links that promote healthy eating. Tel: 416-596-0857. Website: www.dietitians.ca

The Eating Disorder Resource Centre of British Columbia (EDRCBC) provides educational, referral, and research services to people struggling with disordered eating, including a resource counselor help line. Website: www.disorderedeating.ca/default

Eating Disorder Services is located in New Zealand and offers a range of services for people with eating disorders, their friends and family, schools, universities, community groups, and healthcare professionals. Website: www.eatingdisorders.org.nz/

Eating Disorders Association (EDA) provides information and help on all aspects of eating disorders. Website: www.edauk.com/default.htm

The Eating Disorders Association Inc. (QLD) in Queensland, Australia, aims to support all people affected by eating disorders, to raise community awareness about the prevalence and seriousness of these disorders, and to work toward the prevention of eating disorders. Website: www.uq.net.au/eda/documents/start.html

The Eating Disorders Foundation of Victoria (EDFV) in Australia supports those whose lives are affected by eating disorders. Website: http://www.eatingdisorders.org.au/

Eating Disorder Referral and Information Center (EDReferral) is a comprehensive database of professionals offering services to those who suffer from an eating disorder. Website: www.EDReferral.com

Family and Friends Against Disordered Eating (FADE) is an organization that includes sufferers, parents, friends, professionals, and concerned citizens who draw attention to the needs of all individuals affected by eating disorders. Tel: 416-665-9722 Ext 3. Website: www.fade-on.ca

National Association to Advance Fat Acceptance (NAAFA) works to eliminate discrimination based on body size. Website: www.naafa.org

The **National Eating Disorder Information Centre (NEDIC)** provides information and resources on eating disorders and weight preoccupation. Tel: 416-340-4156. Fax: (416) 340-4736. Website: www.nedic.ca

National Eating Disorders Association (NEDA) is the largest not-for-profit organization in the United States working to prevent eating disorders and provide treatment referrals. Tel: 206-382-3587. Website: www.edap.org

National Eating Disorders Screening Program (NEDSP) is the first large-scale screening program for eating disorders. E-mail: isp@mentalhealthscreening.org

The Quebec Association for Assistance to Persons Suffering from Anorexia Nervosa and Bulimia (ANEB Quebec) helps those whose lives are touched by an eating disorder. Tel: 514-630-0907 or 800-630-0907. Website: www.anebquebec.com

Sheena's Place provides support programs for people with eating disorders and their families based on self-referral. Tel: 416-927-8900. Fax: 416-927-8844. Website: www.sheenasplace.org/

The Society for Adolescent Medicine (SAM) is a multidisciplinary organization of professionals committed to improving the physical and psychosocial health and well-being of all adolescents. Tel: (816) 224-8010. Website: www.adolescenthealth.org

Websites
English Language
Canadian Health Network (CHN) provides information on how to stay healthy and prevent disease. Website: www.canadian-health-network.ca

Something Fishy website on eating disorders has resources of all kinds, including information and online support. Website: www.somethingfishy.org

French Language
www.noah-health.org
www.miata.be

Spanish Language
www.nlm.nih.gov/medlineplus/Spanish/eatingdisorders.html
www.soyunica.gov/mybody/bodyimage/eatingdisorders.aspx
www.nationaleatingdisorders.org/p.asp?WebPage_ID=457&Profile_ID=69476

Hospitals and Clinics
United States of America
California
Lucile Packard Children's Hospital
Eating Disorders Program
Adolescent Medicine
1174 Castro Street, Suite 250
Mountain View, CA 94040
Tel: 650-694-0600
Fax: 650-694-0610
Website: www.lpch.org/

UCLA Neuropsychiatric Institute
Adolescent Eating Disorders Program
760 Westwood Plaza
Los Angeles, CA 90024
Tel: 310-825-0511
Website: www.npi.ucla.edu/

Colorado
The Children's Hospital Denver
The Eating Disorders Program
1056 E. 19th Avenue
Denver, CO 80218
Tel: 303-861-6131
Fax: 303-837-2962
Website: www.thechildrenshospital.org/

Massachusetts
Children's Hospital Boston
Eating Disorders Program
333 Longwood Avenue
Boston, MA 02115
Tel: 617-355-7178
Fax: 617-232-1851
Website: www.childrenshospital.org

Harvard Eating Disorders Center
55 Fruit Street
YAW 6900
Boston, MA 02114
Tel: 617-726-8470
Website: www.hedc.org

New York
The Children's Hospital at Montefiore
3415 Bainbridge Avenue, 3rd Floor
Bronx, NY 10467
Tel: 718-741-2450
Website: www.montefiore.org/

**North-Shore Long Island Jewish
Health System**
270-05 76th Avenue
New Hyde Park, New York 11040
Tel: 516-470-7000
Website: www.northshorelij.com/

Ohio
Cincinnati Children's Hospital
3333 Burnet Avenue
Cincinnati, OH 45229-3039
Tel: 513-636-8602
Fax: 513-636-7844
Website: www.cincinnatichildrens.org/

Canada
Alberta
Provincial Contact
Provincial Eating Disorder Coordinator
Tel: 403-297-2026

Alberta Children's Hospital
Calgary Eating Disorder Program
Tel: 403-943-7700
Website:
www.calgaryhealthregion.ca/eatingdis

University of Alberta Hospital
Edmonton Eating Disorder Program
Tel: 780-407-6239
Website: www.cha.ab.ca

British Columbia
British Columbia Children's Hospital
Eating Disorders Program
4480 Oak Street
Vancouver, BC V6H 3V4
Tel: 604-875-2424
Website: www.cw.bc.ca

Manitoba
University of Manitoba
Child & Adolescent Psychiatry Eating
Disorders Service
University of Manitoba
Winnipeg, MB R3T 2N2
Tel: 204-474-8880
Website: www.umanitoba.ca

Newfoundland
Adolescent Medicine Team
Janeway Child Health Centre
300 Prince Philip Drive
St. John's, NL A1B 3V6
Tel: 709-777-4963
Fax: 709-777-4726

Nova Scotia
IWK Health Centre
5850/5980 University Avenue
PO Box 9700
Halifax, NS B3K 6R8
Tel: 902-470-8375
Fax: 902-470-8937
Website: www.iwk.nshealth.ca

Ontario
**Bulimia and Anorexia Nervosa Association
(BANA)**
300 Cabana Road East
Windsor, ON N9G 1A3
Tel: 519-969-2112
Fax: 519-969-0227
Website: www.bana.ca

**Centre for Addiction & Mental Health
(CAMH)**
Concurrent Eating Disorder & Substance
Abuse Program
Addiction Program
250 College Street
Toronto, ON M5T 1R8
Tel: 416-535-8501 Ext 6878
Fax: 416-595-6399
Website: www.camh.net

**Children's Hospital of Eastern Ontario
(CHEO)**
401 Smyth Road
Ottawa, ON K1H 8L1
Tel: 613-737-7600
Fax: 613-738-4854
Website: www.cheo.on.ca

Homewood Health Care
150 Delphi Street
Guelph, ON M1E 6K9
Tel: 519-824-1010 Ext 292
Fax: 519-824-0995
Website: www.homewoodcentre.com

The Hospital for Sick Children
The Eating Disorders Program
555 University Avenue
Toronto, ON M5G 1X8
Tel: 416-813-7195
Fax: 416-813-7867
Website: www.sickkids.ca

London Health Sciences Centre
800 Commissioners Road East
London, ON M6A 4G5
Tel: 519-646-6100
Website: www.lhsc.on.ca

McMaster Children's Hospital
1200 Main Street West
Hamilton, ON L8N 3Z5
Tel: 905-521-2100
Fax: 905-521-2100
Website:
www.mcmasterchildrenshospital.ca

**Niagara Eating Disorder Outpatient Program
(NEDOP)**
Port Colborne Hospital Site
260 Sugarloaf Street
Port Colborne, ON L3K 2N7
Tel: 905-834-4501
Fax: 905-834-3002
Website: www.newportcentre.on.ca

North York General Hospital
The Eating Disorder Program
4001 Leslie Street
Willowdale, ON M2K 1E1
Tel: 416-756-6495
Fax: 416-756-6740
Website: www.nygh.on.ca

Southlake Regional Health Centre
595 Davis Drive
Newmarket, ON L3Y 2P9
Tel: 905-895-4521
Fax: 905-830-5972
Website: www.southlakeregional.org/

**University Health Network: The Toronto
General Hospital**
Eating Disorder Program
200 Elizabeth Street
Toronto, ON M5G 2C4
Tel: 416-340-3041
Website: www.uhn.ca/tgh/index.asp

Quebec
Hospital Sainte-Justine
3175, chemin de la Côte-Ste-Catherine
Montreal, QC H3T 1C5
Tel: 514-345-4721
Fax: 514-345-4778
Website: www.hsj.ca

Montreal Children's Hospital
1 Place Alexis Nihon
3400 de Maisonneuve Blvd. West
Montreal, QC H3Z 3B8
Tel: 514-934-4846 or 866-934-4846
Fax: 514-939-3551
Website: www.thechildren.com

References

American Dietetic Association and Dietitians of Canada. *Manual of Clinical Dietetic.* 6th ed. Chicago, IL: American Dietetic Association, 2000.

American Psychiatric Association. *Diagnostic and Statistical Manual of Mental Disorders.* 4th ed. Washington, DC: American Psychiatric Association, 1994.

American Psychiatric Association. *Practice Guidelines for the Treatment of Patients with Eating Disorders.* Arlington, VA: American Psychiatric Association, 2000.

Anderson-Fye EP, Becker AE. Sociocultural aspects of eating disorders. In Thompson K, ed. *Handbook of Eating Disorders and Obesity.* Hoboken, NJ: John Wiley and Sons, 2004.

Beatty D. Normal healthy eating for teens. *National Eating Disorder Information Centre Bulletin.*1994;9(2).

Becker AE, Keel P, Anderson-Fe EP, Thomas JJ. Genes and/or jeans?: Genetic and socio-cultural contributions to risk for eating disorders. *J Addict Dis.* 2004;23(3):81-103.

Bodysense: A positive body image initiative for female athletes. Available at: www.bodysense.ca

Brewerton TD. Bulimia in children and adolescents. *Child Adolesc Psychiatr Clin N Am.* 2002;1(2):237-56.

Bryant-Waugh R, Lask B. *Eating disorders: A Parent's Guide.* London, UK: Penguin, 1999.

Bryant-Waugh R, Lask B. *Eating Disorders: A Parents' Guide.* rev. ed. Hove, UK and New York, NY: Brunner-Routledge, 2004.

Bulik C. Genetic and biological risk factors. In: Thompson K, ed. *Handbook of Eating Disorders and Obesity.* Hoboken, NJ: John Wiley and Sons, 2004.

Bulik CM, Tozzi F. Contemporary thinking about the role of genes and environment in eating disorders. *Epidemiol Psychiatr Soc.* 2004;13(2):91-98.

Calgary Health Region Website. Available at: www.crha-health.ab.ca
Colahan M, Senior R. Family patterns in eating disorders: Going round in circles, getting nowhere fasting. In: Szmukler G, Dare C, Treasure J, eds. *Handbook of Eating Disorders: Theory, Treatment and Research.* Chichester, UK and New York, NY: John Wiley and Sons, 1995:243-57.

Crisp AH. *Anorexia Nervosa: Let Me Be.* London, UK: Academic, 1980.

Davis R, et al. *The Road to Recovery: A Manual for Participants in the Psycho-education Group for Bulimia Nervosa.* Toronto, ON: The Toronto Hospital, Toronto General Division, 1989.

Dunkely TL, Wertheim EH, Paxton SJ. Examination of a model of multiple sociocultural influences on adolescent girls' body dissatisfaction and dietary restraint. *Adolescence.* 2001;36:265-79.

Eliot A. Group coleadership: A new role for parents of adolescents with anorexia and bulimia nervosa. *International Journal of Group Psychotherapy.* New York, NY: Guildford Publications, 1990.

Erickson, EH. *Identity: Youth and Crisis.* New York: Norton, 1968.

Fisher M. The course and outcome of eating disorders in adults and adolescents: A review. *Adolescent Medicine: State of the Art Reviews.* 2003;149-58.

Fisman S. Pharmacotherapy of early onset eating disorders, child and adolescent. *Psychopharmacology News.* New York, NY: Guildford Publications, 2003.

Fraleigh J, Schmelefske J, Henderson K, Pinhas L. *Why Weight? A Psychoeducational Program for Teens with Eating Disorders and their Families*. Newmarket, ON: Southlake Regional Health Centre, 1999.

Garner D, Garfinkel P. *Handbook of Treatment for Eating Disorders*. 2nd ed. New York, NY: The Guilford Press, 1997.

Garner D, Garfinkel P. *Handbook of Psychotherapy for Anorexia Nervosa and Bulimia*. New York: The Guilford Press, 1997.

Garner DM, Vitousek KM, Pike KM. Reasoning error categories among eating disordered people. In: Garner DM, Garfinkel PE, eds. *Handbook of Treatment for Eating Disorders*. 2nd ed. New York, NY: The Guilford Press, 1997.

Gleaves DH, Miller KJ, Williams TL, Summers SA. Eating disorders: An overview. In: Miller KJ and Mizes JS, eds. *Comparative Treatments for Eating Disorders*. New York, NY: Springer Publishing, 2000.

Golden NH. Eating disorders in adolescents and their sequelae. *Best Pract Res Clin Obstet Gynaecol*. 2003;17(1):57-73.

Golden NH, Katzman DK, Kreipe RE, Stevens SL, Sawyer SM, Rees J, Nicholls D, Rome ES. Eating disorders in adolescents: Position paper of the Society for Adolescent Medicine. *J Adolesc Health*. 2003;33(6):496-503.

Goodwin RA, Mickalide, AD. Parent-to-parent support in anorexia nervosa and bulimia. *Children's Health Care*. 1985.

Gowers S, Bryant-Waugh R. Management of child and adolescent eating disorders: The current evidence base and future directions. *J Child Psychol Psychiatry*. 2004;4(1):63-83.

Greenspan FS, Gardner DG. *Basic & Clinical Endocrinolog*. 6th ed. San Francisco, CA: Lang Medical Books/McGraw-Hill Medical Publishing Division, 2001.

Gusella J, Casey S. A Review of Evidence-Based Treatments for Children and Adolescents with Eating Disorders. *The Canadian Child Psychiatry Review*. 2004;4(1):63-83.

Heinmaa M, Katzman DK, Pinhas L, Agar P. *Alternative Predictors of Inpatient Readmission in Adolescents with Eating Disorders*. Orlando, FL: 2004 International Conference on Eating Disorders, 2004.

Herbold NH, Frates SE. Update of nutrition guidelines for the teen: Trends and concerns. *Current Opinion in Pediatrics*. 2000;12:303-09.

Herrin, M. *Nutrition Counseling in the Treatment of Eating Disorders*. New York, NY: Taylor and Francis, 2003.

Herrin M, Matsumoto N. *The Parents' Guide to Childhood Eating Disorders*. New York, NY: Henry Holt and Company, 2002.

Jasper K. *Reflections on Genes and Eating Disorders*. Toronto, ON: National Eating Disorder Information Centre Bulletin, 2003.

Jones JM, Bennett S, Olmsted MP, Lawson ML, Rodin G. Disordered eating attitudes and behaviours in teenaged girls: A school-based study. *Canadian Medical Association Journal*. 2001;165(5):547-52.

Joffe A, Blythe MJ, eds. Biologic and psychosocial growth and development. *Adolescent Medicine: State of the Art Reviews*. 2003;14(2):231-62.

Kaplan AS. Psychological treatments for anorexia nervosa: A review of published studies and promising new directions. *Can. J of Psychiatry*. 2002;47:235-42.

Kaplan AS, Woodside B. *Genes and Eating Disorders: Unravelling the Mystery*. Toronto, ON: National Eating Disorder Information Centre Bulletin, 2003.

Katchadourian H. *The Biology of Adolescence*. San Francisco, CA: W. H. Freeman and Company, 1977.

Katzman DK, Golden NH, Neumark-Sztainer D, Yager J, Strober M. From prevention to prognosis: Clinical research update on adolescent eating disorders. *Pediatr Res*. 2000;47(6):709-12.

Katzman DK. Osteoporosis in anorexia nervosa: A brittle future? *Curr Drug Targets CNS Neurol Disord*. 2003;2(1):11-15.

Katzman DK. Anorexia nervosa in adolescents: Unique medical complications. *Int J Eat Disord* (in press).

Kerem NC, Katzman DK. Brain structure and function in adolescents with anorexia nervosa. *Adolesc Med.* 2003;14(1):109-18.

Keys A, Brozek J, Henschel A, Mickelsen O, Taylor HL. *The Biology of Human Starvation.* Minneapolis, MN: University of Minnesota Press, 1950.

Kohn M, Golden NH. Eating disorders in children and adolescents: Epidemiology, diagnosis and treatment. *Paediatr Drugs.* 2001;3(2):91-99.

Laliberte M. *Making Changes: A Manual for Group-Based Cognitive Behavior Therapy for Eating Disorders.* Hamilton, ON: St. Joseph's Hospital, 2004.

Larson DR. *The American Dietetic Association's Complete Food & Nutrition Guide.* Chicago, IL: The American Dietetic Association, 1996.

Lask B. Aetiology. In Lask B, Bryant-Waugh R, eds. *Anorexia Nervosa and Related Eating Disorders in Childhood and Adolescence.* East Sussex, UK: Psychology Press, 2000.

Lask B, Bryant-Waugh R, eds. *Anorexia Nervosa and Related Eating Disorders in Childhood and Adolescence.* East Sussex, UK: Psychology Press, 2000.

Levenkron S. *Anatomy of Anorexia.* New York, NY: W.W. Norton, 2000.

Litt IF. *Evaluation of the Adolescent Patient.* Philadelphia, PA: Hanley & Belfus, 1990.

Lewis HL, MacQuire MP. Review of a group for parents of anorexics. *Journal of Psychiatric Research.* 1985:19 (2-3):453-58.

Lock J, Le Grange D, Agras WS, Dare C. Chapter 1: Information and background information on anorexia nervosa. In: Lock J, ed. *Treatment Manual for Anorexia Nervosa: A Family Based Approach.* New York, NY: The Guilford Press, 2001.

Macdonald M. Bewildered, blamed and broken-hearted: Parents' views of anorexia nervosa. In: Lask B, Bryant-Waugh R, eds. *Anorexia Nervosa and Related Disorders in Childhood and Adolescence.* 2nd ed. East Sussex, UK: Psychology Press, 2000.

Maine M. *Body Wars: Making Peace with Women's Bodies.* Carlsbad, CA: Gurze Books, 2000.

Malloy JM, Cheney D, Cormier GM. Interagency collaboration and the transition to adulthood for students with emotional or behavioral disabilities. *Education & Treatment of Children: Special Severe Behavior Disorders of Children and Youth.* 1998;21(3):303-20.

Marcus MD, Kalarchian MA. Binge eating in children and adolescents. *Int J Eat Disord.* 2003;34 Suppl:S47-57.

McCreary Centre Society. Adolescent health survey II: Province of British Columbia. Vancouver, BC: The McCreary Centre Society, 1999.

McKinley R. Life at the end of the tunnel. *Listener.* September 7, 2002.

McVey GL, Davis R, Tweed S, Shaw B. An evaluation of a school-based program designed to improve body image satisfaction, global self-esteem, and eating attitudes and behaviors: A replication study. *International Journal of Eating Disorders.* 2004;36:1-11.

McVey GL, Lieberman M, Voorberg N, Wardrope D, Blackmore E, Tweed S. Replication of a prevention program designed to reduce disordered eating: Is a life skills approach sufficient for all middle school students? *Eating Disorders: Journal of Treatment and Prevention.* 2003;11:187-96.

McVey GL, Lieberman M, Voorberg N, Wardrope D, Blackmore E. School-based peer support groups: A new approach to the prevention of eating disorders. *Eating Disorders: Journal of Treatment and Prevention.* 2003;11:169-86.

McVey G, Tweed S, Blackmore E. Dieting among preadolescent and young adolescent females. *Canadian Medical Association Journal.* 2004;170(10):1559-61.

McVey GL, Tweed S, Blackmore E. Correlates of weight loss and muscle gaining behaviors in 10-14 year old males and females. *Preventive Medicine.* 2004;40:1-9.

Melina V, Davis B, Harrison V. *Becoming Vegetarian.* Toronto, ON: Macmillan Canada, 1994.

Miller W, Rollnick S, Conforti K. *Motivational Interviewing: Preparing People for Change.* 2nd ed. New York: The Guilford Press, 2002.

The Minister of Health Canada. The *Vitality Approach: A Guide for Leaders.* Ottawa, ON: The Minister of Health Canada , 2000.

National Eating Disorder Information Centre. *An Introduction to Food and Weight Problems.* Toronto, ON: University Health Network: Toronto General Hospital, 2003. Available at: www.nedic.on.ca

National Eating Disorder Information Centre. *Understanding and Overcoming an Eating Disorder.* Toronto, ON: University Health Network: Toronto General Hospital, 2003. Available at: www.nedic.on.ca

Neinstein LS. *Adolescent Health Care, A Practical Guide.* 4th ed. Philadelphia, PA: Lippincott, Williams & Wilkins, 2002.

Nielsen S, Bara-Carril N. Family, burden of care and social consequences. In Treasure J, Schmidt U, van Furth E, eds. *Handbook of Eating Disorders.* 2nd ed. Chichester, UK: John Wiley & Sons, 2003.

Patton GC, Johnson-Sabine E, Wood K, Mann AH, Wakeling A. Abnormal eating attitudes in London schoolgirls: A prospective epidemiological study: Outcome at twelve month follow-up. *Psychological Medicine.* 1990;20:383-94.

Patton GC, Selzer R, Coffey C, Carlin JB, Wolfe R. Onset of adolescent eating disorders: Population based cohort study over 3 years. *British Medical Journal.* 1999;318:765-68.

Polivy J, Herman CP. Causes of eating disorders. *Annual Review of Psychology.* 2002;53:187-213.

Powers PS, Santana CA. Childhood and adolescent anorexia nervosa. *Child Adolesc Psychiatr Clin N Am.* 2002;11(2):219-35.

Prochaska J, Johnson S, Lee P. The transtheoretical model of behavior change. In: Shumaker SA, Schron EB, eds. *The Handbook of Health Behavior Change.* 2nd ed. New York, NY: Springer Publishing, 1998:59-84.

Prochaska J, Norcross J, DiClemente D. *Changing for Good.* New York, NY: Perennial Currents/Harper Collins, 1995.

Quality School Health. Canadian Association for Health, Physical Education, Recreation and Dance. Available at: www.cahperd.ca.

Reder P, McClure M, Jolley A. *Family Matters: Interfaces between Child and Adult Mental Health.* New York, NY: Routledge, 2000.

Rome ES, Ammerman S, Rosen DS, Keller RJ, Lock J, et al. Children and adolescents with eating disorders: The state of the art. *Pediatrics.* 2003;111(1):e98-108.

Rosen DS. Eating disorders in children and young adolescents: Etiology, classification, clinical features, and treatment. *Adolesc Med.* 2003;14(1):49-59.

Sargent J. Teaching house staff about eating disorders. *Pediatric Annals.* 1992;21:720-27.

Satter, E. *Secrets of Feeding a Healthy Family.* Madison, WI: Kelcy Press, 1999.

Sawin KJ, Cox AW, Metzger SG, Horsley, JW, Harrigan MP, Deaton A, Thompson EC. Transition planning for youth with chronic conditions: An interdisciplinary process. *National Academies of Practice Forum: Issues in Interdisciplinary Care.* 1999;1(3):183-96.

Schene A. (1990). Objective and subjective dimensions of family burden: Towards an integrative framework for research. *Social Psychiatry and Psychiatric Epidemiology.* 1990;25:289-97.

Schneider M. Bulimia nervosa and binge-eating disorder in adolescents. *Adolesc Med.* 2003;14(1):119-31.

Seaver A, McVey G, Fullerton Y, Stratton L. (1997). *Every BODY is a Somebody: An Active Learning Program to Promote Healthy Body Image, Positive Self-esteem, Healthy Eating and an Active Lifestyle for Adolescent Females: Teachers Guide.* Brampton, ON: Body Image Coalition of Peel, 1997. Available at: www.bodyimagecoalition.org

Seid RP. *Never Too Thin: Why Women Are at War with Their Bodies.* New York, NY: Prentice Hall Press, 1989.

Sharkey-Orgnero MI. Anorexia nervosa: A qualitative analysis of parent's perspectives on recovery. *Eating Disorders: The Journal of Treatment and Prevention.* 1999;7(2):123-41.

Shelley R, ed. *Anorexics on Anorexia.* London, UK: Jessica Kingsley Publishers, 2000.

Siegal M, et al. *Surviving an Eating Disorder: Strategies for Family and Friends.* New York, NY: HarperCollins, 1997.

Smolak L, Levine M. *The Developmental Psychopathology of Eating Disorders: Implications for Research, Prevention, and Treatment.* Hillsdale, NJ: Lawrence Erlbaum Associates, 1996.

Society for Nutrition Education. Weight realities division, 2003. Available at: www.sne.org

Szmukler G. From family 'burden' to caregiving. *Psychiatric Bulletin.* 1996;20:449-51.

Strober M, Freeman R, Morell W. The long-term course of severe anorexia nervosa in adolescents: Survival analysis of recovery, relapse and outcome predictors over 10-15 years in a prospective study. *Int J Eat Disord.* 1997;22(4):339-60.

Treasure J. *Anorexia Nervosa: A Survival Guide for Families, Friends and Sufferers.* East Sussex, UK: Psychology Press, 1997.

Treasure J, Murphy T, Szmukler G, Todd G, Gavan K, Joyce J. The experience of caregiving for severe mental illness: A comparison between anorexia nervosa and psychosis. *Social Psychiatry and Psychiatric Epidemiology.* 2001;36:343-47.

Vandereycken W. The families of patients with an eating disorder. In Brownell K, Dare C, eds. *Eating Disorders and Obesity: A Comprehensive Handbook.* London: The Guilford Press, 1995:219-23.

Vandereycken W, Kog E, Vanderlinden J. *The Family Approach to Eating Disorders.* New York, NY: PMA Publishing, 1989.

Vitousek K, Watson S, Wilson GT. Enhancing motivation for change in treatment-resistant eating disorders. *Clinical Psychology Review.* 1998;18(4):391-420.

Washington State Department of Health Available at: www.faculty.washington.edu/jrees/adolescentnutrition.html

Watzlawick P, Weakland J, Fisch R. *Change: Principles of Problem Formation and Resolution.* New York, NY: W. W. Norton, 1974.

Wood D, Flowers P, and Black D. Should parents take charge of their child's eating disorder? Some preliminary findings and suggestions for future research. *International Journal of Psychiatry in Clinical Practice.* 1998;2(4):295-301.

Young J, Klosko J. *Reinventing Your Life.* New York, NY: Plume Books, 1994.

Acknowledgments

We want to express our gratitude and admiration to the authors, our treasured colleagues, for contributing to this book. We thank you for sharing your hard work, dedication and expertise. We would also like to acknowledge the members of the larger interdisciplinary team in the Eating Disorders Program at The Hospital for Sick Children for their tireless commitment to helping children and adolescents with eating disorders and their families.

To our publisher, Bob Dees, we thank him for his insight and guidance, and to our editor, Bob Hilderley, for his creative approach and thoughtful suggestions. It was a pleasure to work with you both!

This book was completed in large part due to the hard work and patience of Ursula Pajak and Heather Graham. We could not have completed this project without their unrelenting patience, perseverance and support.

We would like to acknowledge the people who have supported us throughout our careers: Drs. Hugh O'Brodovich, Eudice Goldberg, Abel Ickowicz, Joseph Beitchman and Brenda Toner. A special thanks to Judy Burns for her unwavering commitment and support. We would also like to acknowledge the work of John Schmelefske and Jill Fraleigh, whose clinical knowledge and innovative spirit influenced this book.

Finally, we would like to pay a special tribute to our patients and families in the Eating Disorders Program. You inspire us to continue to do our best. You have taught us the importance of an open mind and a caring heart. Thank you for teaching us so much.

Index